Tough Love

A Stutterer's Survival Kit

by

Shane Chapa

Chapa Communications
toughlovestutter@gmail.com
24 W. Camelback Rd., ste. A-218
Phoenix, AZ 85013

Photos Courtesy of the Author
Robert L. McCullough, Editor
butterflybeachmedia@gmail.com

ISBN: 9798602444063

Copyright © 2020 Chapa Communications

All rights reserved under international and Pan-American Copyright Conventions. Published in the United States by
Chapa Communications, Phoenix, Arizona
No part of this publication may be reproduced, stored in any format or system, or transmitted at any time of by any means, electronic, mechanical, photocopying, recording, or otherwise without the expressed prior permission of the copyright holder.
This book is sold subject to the condition that it shall not by way of trade or otherwise be circulated without the publisher's prior consent in any form of binding or cover other than that in which is it published

Cataloging-in-Publication Data

Chapa, Shane, 1978-
Tough Love – A Stutterer's Survival Kit / by Shane Chapa
ISBN 9798602444063
 1. Psychology. 2. Memoir. 3. Self-help. 4. Speech Therapy   Chapa Communications 2020.

Shane Chapa

This book is dedicated to anyone
who has ever loved a stutterer.

Tough Love

Introduction

Trust me on this: This book is not for everyone. As a matter of fact, some will find it offensive and others will find it blasphemy to the "I'm special" self-image paradigm of stuttering they exist in.

If I come off as irreverent or sarcastic...*mea culpa*. It won't be the first time. That doesn't mean I'm insensitive or judgmental in any way. I'm not really trying to come off like a complete A-hole here, because I'm well aware that we all walk our own paths and sometimes have to hack our way through the jungle just to make any progress on our individual journeys.

My personal journey has required more than my fair share of inner strength, courage and an uncompromising belief that a man's determination to pursue his individual purpose is the only thing by which he can be defined.

I'm going to be speaking to you bluntly here, perhaps more in-your-face than anyone ever has. You see, I really don't care if your feelings get hurt or if you've got a closet full of stuttering convention t-shirts splattered with some tritely "positive" messaging. What I *do* care about is that the reality you create for yourself is one of victory, empowerment, and self-worth.

Look, you can live as a handicapped, disassociated member of an increasingly self-pitying society or you can be happy, healthy and live a purposeful, self-determined life. I want you to do just that with empathy, action, and the power of a wise ruler of his or her own domain.

That's why I'm writing this book.

I have searched for meaningful self-help books for stutterers and they're hard to find. Know why? Because people who stutter want a complete cure, and they don't have the patience for anything less. I've joined a few stuttering groups online and have even done my best to support a few organizations, but I'm just not feeling it. I can't handle one more "tell me about your hardest moment as a stutterer." Here's a news flash: every moment is fucking hard.

Those people who have had successful careers, amazing social lives, and full lives as a stutterer aren't online. They're out there, doing things and living with their stutter, not *as* a stutterer.

So right now, you're a stutterer. And it's possible that at some point, you'll figure out how to speak fluently and that'll be terrific. But now, whenever you open your mouth unpredictable speech patterns erupt from the storm inside your head. How you navigate this storm is up to you.

I can talk like a robot, slowly pronounce every syllable and speak more fluently. Practicing these exercises is a good idea to gain better motor control and muscle memory, but you are not a robot and your memory is awash with all the battles with stuttering that you've lost. Stuttering has defeated you because you've fought it. You've been fighting an invisible opponent and now you're so tired of swinging at nothing that it's just easier to beat yourself up. You've been fighting so hard to be a non-stutterer for so long you no longer have any idea who you are.

Maybe you're a self-loathing Mr. Nice Guy or Girl who can't succeed or find love and friendship and you wake up every morning accepting what you believe is your perpetual state of mediocrity. This is not the fault of the stutter or any neurological phenomenon, the kids who bullied you, the inpatient cashier who sighs annoyingly, or a society that doesn't understand what it's like to stutter. This "mediocrity" perception is of your own creation. You've done this to yourself, you've felt sorry for yourself and you've spent more time wallowing than swimming.

I get it, folks. At times, it really sucks. You probably got beat up in bathrooms at school, were mimicked, laughed at, belittled and convinced you were worthless. But, you are your own person and your paradigm, what you believe about yourself, is truly up to you.

I've been through it, in it, under it, around it, and it kicked my ass up and down both sides of Hard Knocks Avenue. It's easy to be there and just be a victim. As a stutterer, accepting that victimhood might be the easier choice.

But what if it's not the stutter? What if everybody has to deal with the same inner turmoil, but we blame the stutter because it gets us extra attention and sympathy? What if our stutter is actually our strength, a leg up on life, and we don't realize it. It's all about perspective and framing things in such a way that stuttering works *for you* and not against you.

Years ago, I dated a woman named Jessica. She was a nurse who took care of people dying from cancer. She had a very realistic outlook on life. She was awesome, made even more so because she clearly adored me. (I broke up with her because I felt like "Roger Rabbit," but we'll get into that later.) I came home from work one day with a huge cut on my arm. As a seasoned construction worker, I felt that shop rags and duct tape were appropriate for the situation. As a tenured nurse, however, she thought I was an idiot. She forced me into the bathroom, sat me on the toilet, and properly dressed the wound.

As I sat there, pretending that ripping the duct tape off my hairy arm didn't hurt, she asked me why I didn't wear more protective equipment. I worked with glass, cuts were inevitable, and protective equipment made common sense. So did her question. I said, "Chicks dig scars" with a wink, expecting her to melt into my valiant, rugged arms, intoxicated by my virile masculine charms. Instead, she rolled her eyes, looked at me like I was an idiot and said, "Chicks don't dig the scar; they dig the story."

Whoa. There was an epiphany. It was one of those moments when your ego gets knocked on its ass and you learn something. She was right, the scar grabs attention and initiates curiosity, just like a stutter does, but the attention and curiosity depend entirely upon the story.

If you keep reading, I just might knock *your ego* on its ass.

"I've had a stuttering problem my whole life. I'm just cool with it now."

~Shaquille O'Neal

1.
Why Fear?

Not all storms come to disrupt your life.
Some come to clear your path.

Why are you so shy and scared of the world? Because you stutter. Why am I so fearless and outgoing? Because I stutter. That's my choice. You can make your own. You can choose fear...or you can choose to be fear*less*.

It's a simple decision, and one that only you can make. Your personality, your drive, and your self-esteem will determine whether your story is one of courage or fear, and if your scar is one of a warrior or a victim.

I met a man who served in Iraq as a Marine. He had a glass eye with the globe and anchor etched on it. He'd lost his eye in an IED explosion during a convoy. Is he a victim? He suffered wounds at the hands of another person. He was permanently disfigured in the course of doing his job. Sounds like he's a victim, doesn't it? Could he live as a victim? Yes, he could get a glass eye that matches his other eye and try to look like everyone else. He could undoubtedly earn sympathy from every American for the pain he's endured. But does he identify himself as a victim? Hell no! He proudly wears the symbol of his beloved Marine Corps as his scar, looks completely different from anyone else with the same injury, and doesn't give a shit what anyone has to say about it. He's a hero, not a victim. He's a Marine, not a victim. He's a badass, not a victim. He is a *survivor*, not a victim.

I'm not comparing stuttering to war. I'm comparing the mindset of someone who wants to fit in to someone else who is proud not to. I spent most of my life stuttering and trying to fit in, and I did a damned good job of it. I personally didn't know anyone else who stuttered until I was in my 30s, so this has always been a solo "combat mission" and honestly, I'm thankful for that.

I spent decades trying to hide my stutter. All I ever wanted to be was a non-stutterer and to be graciously accepted into the non-stuttering world. You know what I learned? People who do *not* stutter are just as frightened of public speaking, approaching a member of the opposite sex, and enduring job interviews as we stutterers are. They're actually *more* scared! The bottom line is that if you grow up as a person who is in no way different from anyone else, your biggest fear is to stand out in a crowd or be different.

As a stutterer, I've always stood out. I've always caught the attention of anyone within earshot. "Different" is all I've ever known. So, if the greatest fear of the general population is a stutterer's default setting, what are *you* afraid of when speaking or approaching anyone? Here's the dirty little secret that you and I both know: You're afraid that you will stutter. You're afraid your mouth will get locked in a weird position, your eyes will roll to the back of your head and you'll block for so long you'll forget what you were gonna say in the first place.

But that's not even stuttering. That's you fighting the stutter. That's you trying to stop a tsunami by standing in front of it (never a good idea). You can reframe this. Don't fight it. Don't hate it. Just treat it as a glorious battle scar with its own story of courage and perseverance. You'll find that your stutter is not your enemy, that it's a scar that only you are allowed to define, whose story only you truly know. At the end of the day, what others learn about your scar is entirely up to you. Make it a great story, because the only thing you need to change about yourself is your perspective. How *you* perceive your scar is how others will perceive your stuttering, so wear it proudly.

Tough Love

2.
Roger Rabbiting

Too many people overvalue what they are not and undervalue what they are.
~Malcolm S. Forbes

For the record, I am a completely average guy physically. I'm 5'8', kind of soft around the middle, thinning out on top and tell myself that the greys growing out of my chin are totally badass. I was in good shape during my military years and keep my weight under 170. Today, I have a true "dad bod." That's a body that was once totally ripped-and-fit. I still carry the remnants of an athletic physique, but it's obvious that I wave at the gym as I drive past more often than I go in. I've never been broke but I've never been rich. My income level has generally hovered around the national median for my generational demographic. I can't sing or play any musical instruments, have no artistic talents, and can't cook. I am in no way a ladies man and have nothing that a woman would date me for besides, well just myself.

In spite of my utter lack of personal exceptionalism, my dating and love life has always been abundant. I've dated amazing women, my sex life has always been well above average, and the women with whom I've been involved have been well-adjusted in every respect. But all those potentially lasting relationships ended simply because I was too insecure or felt somehow unworthy of being in a committed relationship. But if notches on a bedpost are your definition of success in romance, the measure of a man, or a gauge of true personal satisfaction, you should put this book down and find something else to read because you've got bigger issues to deal with than your stutter.

I know this because for years, I searched for my own self-worth in the validation of others. Especially validation by the women in my life. Yes, sex is an amazing source of momentary validation as you're awash in dopamine and self-confidence . . . until she rolls over and you start scrolling through your phone like an addict looking for a fix because this one just wore off and if you don't get another moment of affirmation you just might have to face yourself. Perish *that* thought!

~ ~ ~

Jessica was gorgeous inside and out. She had the figure of a swimsuit model, a mature and seductive voice. She was educated, cultured, successful, poised and mentally secure. She knew how sexy she was but placed no self-worth on it. She was all of these things as a result of her genuine self-respect. She was in love with me and treated me very well. I was in the midst of growing pains as an entrepreneur and didn't have much money to spend on her. I was in good shape but not chiseled, and my stutter at that time was still pretty severe. I kept looking for something wrong with her. Otherwise, why would she be with me? In the back of my mind, whenever we walked into a restaurant together, I felt like we must've looked like "Jessica and Roger Rabbit," and I wasn't the sexy half of this couple.

    She wanted to buy a house closer to where I lived and someday—sooner rather than later—move in together. I told her we weren't going to work out; I was honest and straight forward. I told her I thought she was too good for me and I couldn't handle it. She cussed me out and cried. I could hear the authentic pain in her voice as she expressed her feelings towards me. I didn't understand this until years later when the woman I'm now in a long-term healthy relationship with wouldn't let me do the same to her. My current partner dug her heels in when I suggested that it was time for her to move on, that I didn't deserve her, blah, blah, blah. She made it clear that she'd invested meaningful years into our relationship and flat-out refused to let me throw away what we built together.

Crazy, huh? Find a fabulous woman, enjoy a terrific relationship with her, and then—rather than face my own insecurities—jump ship. Bail out. Head for the exit.

That's what I'd done to every woman I've ever been with. I either told them it was too much for me, or my lack of self-esteem extinguished any attraction they had for me and they gave up and just walked away. Jessica loved me because I was a man with a mission. I was obsessed with being self-employed, I was pursuing my dreams, and the fact that I stuttered only made the entire package more attractive to her. She was in love with my passion and drive. She dated men who could speak eloquently, had cash to spend and more time for her, but she was a go-getter herself and she loved the go-getter in me. In her eyes, my stutter was not a negative issue; it was my battle scar. It was a scar that demonstrated perseverance and courage. To me, however, my stutter is what made me unworthy of her. From my perspective at the time, the sacrifices I made to be self-employed were not an expression of any great ambition or passion. They were merely evidence of a handicapped *victim* who had to work harder to succeed than anyone else. My self-worth—my perception of myself—was just below the surface of the water in a gas station toilet, and I was in constant fear that someday someone was going to flush it away.

Perspective can make or break you.

~ ~ ~

I was once engaged to a woman whom I'd met while we were both in the Army. We were reservists and deployed overseas, the perfect setting for a romantic adventure. Two soldiers in a foreign land secretly engaged in a love affair that overcame all odds and moved in together when they returned home. She was tough enough to be a soldier and smart enough to be a scientist. She held a Master's degree from George Washington University in forensic sciences and was honorably discharged from the Army with countless commendations. She loved me too, she stood by me through a lot of hard times, but eventually I managed to wear her down. I was on some sort of misdirected, crazy mission; I had to wear her down, there had to be something wrong with her to be in love with a stutterer. My insecurities and self-hate skewed our romance into a therapist-patient relationship. I had problems and she felt compelled to search for the answers. She tried for years, but I just fell deeper into my own self-loathing to the point that she couldn't be my therapist anymore. She was in the relationship to be my partner, not my parent. One night, my determination to numb the pain with alcohol ended with me exploding with rage and trashing the house. Like any sane woman would, she left.

Talk about a low moment… that's as low as it gets. I did some serious soul-searching and came to the same conclusion I always did when the drinking caused me to lose something I cared about. I drank too much and had a bad temper because it was so frustrating to stutter. My own twisted logic (alcohol does wonders in that department) brought me to believe that she'd lost her feelings for me because I stutter and the obvious corollary was that I was a piece of shit because I stutter.

We'd been quite the social couple. Our weekends had been full of house parties and dinners. She must have introduced me to hundreds of people. Introductions for a stutterer are awkward moments of anxiety riddled with heart murmurs. If you stutter, everyone is going to go wide-eyed in shock, start to fidget, and act overly polite—often to the point of condescension—to you. Unless they're the moronic weird ones who just burst out in laughter. Not really laughter, more of a titter or a stifled guffaw, accompanied by paranoid look in their eyes. If you didn't stutter then, you definitely would later when they inexplicably ask if you're alright because you were just speaking fine and they couldn't understand why. Inconsistent speech patterns seem to irritate people!

She never once felt that way. She introduced me as her man. I was someone she was proud to be with, and she made no excuses for me. Of course, my trepidation at being introduced to strangers was *my* reaction and mine alone. It was all in my head. She was not at all embarrassed that I might stutter upon introduction. But I was petrified of it because my worth as a man was dependent on her attraction to me. I was always writing a disaster movie in the back of my mind: If I freaked those people out, she would feel awkward and would probably fall for that guy who was looking at her and leave me because I STUTTER! See where this is going? Can this rabbit hole of self-defeating bullshit get any deeper?

Anytime I've ever thought a woman would reject me because I stutter, I was lying to myself to cover up another problem. I didn't have to learn to validate myself, improve myself, or grow up and act like a man because I could blame the stutter for everything.

~ ~ ~

The woman I'm with now has been through all of it and has seen the worst of me. She's seen me through a drinking problem, she watched me battle every demon I've had, she's been there as I've completely ignored her needs for years on end, she's stood by while I've toiled in misery and either blamed her or the stutter for my failure to grow up and deal with life as a mature adult. It actually got to the point where I could feel her silent rage when I blamed my stutter for all my problems.

Today, I get it. I understand it now. It gets tiring. It's not the stutter that is the problem; it's the baggage. It's not my fault I stutter, but it's my responsibility to carry my own baggage and not bring others down with me. It's lonely at the bottom and actually rather pathetic. To cause others pain, to take years of their life and give them nothing in return but an ego-filled self-loathing excuse of why you can't grow as a human being is simply selfish and ultimately destructive to everyone involved.

Because I stutter...

What a bullshit excuse for anything.

The bottom line is that you and me, we stutter because we speak disfluently. We generate some very effective relationship destroying issues and narcissistic tendencies because we feel sorry for ourselves.

I can tell these stories many more times and insert a different woman's name. The only common denominator in these stories, however, was me. The issues I had that led to me being the common denominator are low self-esteem, low self-worth and low self-confidence. I hurt women because I felt as if I wasn't good enough for them. The women were all innocent; they didn't

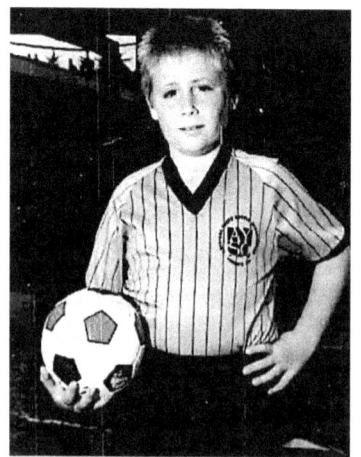

share these feelings at all. Not once was my stutter an issue and not one time was I ever demeaned, put down or criticized for it by any of the terrific women in my life. If anything, the whole stuttering thing was attractive to them. Not the stutter itself, but the courage I had to summon to blaze my own trail in life in spite of the fact that I stuttered. My perspective was flawed. I was the little boy being beat up on the playground because he was different. I'd never really grown up.

Tough Love

3.
Get to Work

If you go into adulthood still stuttering,
you can handle anything. You have been tempered by fire.
~David Seidler

My last job interview was torture. It was summer in Phoenix and I had just moved from Monterey, so I went from a climate where 65° is a warm day to the hottest desert on the continent where 100° weather defines a cold snap. I was drinking gallons of water and couldn't stop sweating if my life depended on it. I had an interview that morning, and I'd just arrived in Phoenix eight hours earlier. I'd had an awesome conversation with the owner of the business several days prior, so I made the trip to meet with him. What I didn't realize—I hadn't checked my voicemail earlier that day—is that he'd already filled the position the day before. So I showed up.

When he told me the bad news, he referred me to a larger shop that was looking to hire a new construction estimator. With nothing to lose, I decided to drop by this other shop. I walked into the office expecting to drop off my resume and leave. By that time, I was running on caffeine and Gatorade, my pants—the only ones I had that weren't a wrinkled mess—were too small for me, cutting off the circulation to my legs, the t-shirt under my dress shirt was soaked, I was stiff and sore from the nonstop 12-hour drive, I hadn't eaten since the day before, I'd just noticed a typo on my resume that I somehow missed after 20 proofreads, and due to all of it contributing to a general feeling of total anxiety, my stutter setting was turned to *just don't talk*. Yes I have stutter settings, and *just don't talk* is in my meter's red zone. The needle was pinned. On a scale of 1-10, I was hitting 14.

I approached the counter filling my lungs with air, tapping my finger on the sheet of paper to get a rhythm going to launch my first word out and clearly said "Good morning, I'm new to the area and would like to drop off my resume for your consideration."

"Of course, here's an application take a seat," she said, pointing to the only chair in the reception area.

Shit, I thought, noticing the chair was right in front of the window being baked by the sun. I sat down and quickly filled the application out. I'd memorized my resume and was able to answer all the questions off the top of my head. I looked up as a man was standing there looking at me as the receptionist handed him my resume. He about-faced and walked down the hall. *That was weird*, I thought as I looked down at the application and then… *No! No! No!* I screamed inside, watching in slow motion as a huge drop of sweat fell down my nose and splatted dead center on the application form. By this time, my back was on fire, sweating profusely to cool itself from the sun baking it. I stood up, sweat dripping down every part of me as I walked towards the receptionist, eager for the moment that I could get out of there kick myself in the ass and change my shirt. Flushed with embarrassment, I handed her the contaminated application as she spoke into her phone with "No problem, he just finished it. I'll see if he can wait." She took the sweat-splattered application without looking at it and said "The commercial department manager would like to speak with you if you can wait around."

Hell no! I was in no way prepared for an interview. The only thing I could feel from the waist down was sweat pooling in my shoes, my shirt was completely soaked, my stutter setting was maxed out, and my nerves were at Defcon 5. "Of course, no problem," I said, scanning the premises for a restroom. I had to get my shit together quick. As I turned toward the hall with the blue triangle on the door at the end of it, the commercial manager walked up to me with his hand outstretched and introduced himself. I am not shy or timid; in fact, I'm actually an extrovert and pretty comfortable in conversation. But this wasn't going to be just any old conversation. This was all about business, about something that mattered. This was going to be me convincing him that I was more capable of doing this job than any straight talking guy who had turned in a resume before me.

How do you do that? If you can't talk straighter, you shoot straighter. I shook his hand firmly and *intentionally stuttered.*

Yes, I intentionally stuttered. I blocked and blinked hard on purpose. I got it out of the way, cleared the air and buried the anxiety clouding my mind. "G-g-g-good morning, I'm Shane."

Like everyone usually does, he froze for a split second to register what was going on, and then gestured with his head for me to follow and led me down a hallway towards his office. This section of the building was cooler. The AC was blasting (yes!) and I slowed my stride to take advantage of it drying my head and neck. I took deep breaths, slowed my heart rate as we entered his office, and I took a seat across from him.

He was a loud, fast-talking guy. Kind of a prick to be honest, but that worked fine for me. As a stutterer, I learned how to handle loudmouth pricks a long time ago. He simultaneously read my resume and complained about everyone who worked there, rattling on about how incompetent they all were. He tossed my resume on his desk, looked me in the eye and vented with, "I need someone who can do this fucking job. Everyone I hire says they can but then has no idea what they're doing and I have to start all over again. They get the software but don't know anything about glass…"

When he was reading my resume, I was going over everything in the room. The vendor books behind him, the software program manuals stacked behind his monitor, and the open blueprints laying on every available surface. Stutterers are masters of situational awareness, and I'm an expert. As children, it's a skill we learn in order to survive; as adults we can use it to thrive.

"On paper you're qualified but you don't have much office experience."

"I-I-I don't," I said, agreeing with him. At this point, I was sure I was done, but sometimes that's the beautiful thing. The pressure was off. No way was I getting this job. So I relaxed; I had no worries because at this point it was just a conversation with a guy hiding his own issues behind an oversize personality. I had field experience. I could read blueprints off the tailgate of a pickup. I'm not a desk jockey, and I suck at Excel. To give you an insight into my prehistoric office skills, I'm actually pecking at a keyboard with two fingers as I write this.

At that moment, sitting in front of this over-the-top guy, I decided to use this impromptu meeting as practice for my next interview, one for which I would be better dressed and better prepared. I was already there, sweaty but enjoying the air conditioning, and I'd already outed my stutter and my nerves were shot from lack of sleep and sheer fatigue, and so...What the hell?...I decided just to be myself, my unpolished, stuttering, not-made-for-the-corporate-world self. Just...Shane.

Once I relaxed, I noticed something. I've noticed it all my life but it came at me in full-color surround-sound 3-D in that moment. *People open up to stutterers.* This guy was telling me his problems and what he needed. I'd said a total of seven words, two of them full-blown blocks and he doesn't give a shit. As usual, I was sitting there terrified that the stuttering police were gonna come get me if I fucked up and, as usual, nobody in that room cared that I stutter. I've learned that non-stutterers often seem so scared of being different that my being different gives them room and a sense of ease. Maybe it's simply because it's obvious I'm not competing with them or trying to get a word in edgewise. My stuttering actually opens up a place of ease in them. (Yes, I'm an obsessive people watcher and probably need some kind of deep, lifelong therapy to correct that little habit.)

So after my interrogator busted me on my total lack of office experience, I said "It takes years to learn a trade, and software takes a week. I already know the product, I can start next week, and in the meantime, I'll just download the tutorial and know the basics by Day One."

This is something we stutterers always do, whether we know it or not. We write love letters instead of proclaiming admiration, we learn to fix things instead of having to explain the problem to someone else, and we order pizza online cause the E in "extra pepperoni" is a killer. We stutterers have been problem solving since we started planning trips to the school lavatory just before our turn came up and we had to orally introduce ourselves to the class.

Ours is a lifetime of "work-arounds." We're a valuable part of the workforce. Our critical thinking and problem solving skills are—out of absolute necessity—honed to perfection. Our situational awareness is a survival tool and our capacity to sidestep unnecessary banter is an art form. A job interview is stressful for anyone; everyone sweats and stutters in that "hot seat," but we actually have an advantage because we're constantly in one, wherever we go. We're in the "hot seat" just ordering dinner in a restaurant, ordering a drink in a loud bar, going to the bank, calling customer service. That "hot seat" is where we live!

There are hundreds of well-known tricks and techniques that are "supposed" to solve the problem, and I've tried them all. But the real solution—instead of reading poetry in front of a mirror or practicing breathing out vowels and letting go of blocks—is to figure out what people need and how you can solve their problem at any given moment. We get so stuck on ourselves and our imperfections that we forget that no one is perfect and everyone needs a survivor on their team. That guy interviewing me? He had a problem, and I was the guy who could solve it. That woman behind the counter? She may have been sent to human resources yesterday because she was impolite to someone. The trick is to stutter with confidence and don't be fazed by how long it takes to finish speaking. That person in front of you just might appreciate someone with thicker skin who can tough it out without being embarrassed or frustrated...or walking away.

4. Perspectives

The happiest stutterers are those who are
willing to stutter in front of others.
~ John Stossel

Perfection. When you find it, let me know because on the planet where I live, there's no such thing.

We think we're up against a perfect world were we don't fit in because we take longer to speak than most people do. The marketplace is about productivity and money. Faster is better. More is better. If you can be productive and add to the bottom line of an organization, you're qualified! If you cannot find a job and you blame it on your stutter, be careful. You may be an unproductive person with no market value blaming your lack of ambition on your stutter. I might sound like an asshole for saying that, but hurting your precious feelings is far better than you not getting it together and having a career.

Here are some painful truths:

There is no financial assistance for you.

There are no handouts for you.

Nobody gives a shit that you stutter.

Your stutter has become a life-defining thing for you because you're at war with it or it's a convenient excuse for whatever you're *not doing*.

Your stutter—no matter how bad *you* may think it is—is perceived by everyone else as nothing more than a minor affliction, even a part of your amazing personality. If it's holding you back or keeping you from doing anything, that's because *you* are letting it control *you*.

Hey, I know that stuttering can suck, especially as a child with no idea what the bigger picture looks like, but for an adult to blame anything on their stutter is a total cop out. I *got* that job. Then I switched departments because that loudmouthed guy was a prick and I then found a better-paying position. I've been to at least ten job interviews in my life. I have stuttered in every one of them and I have never had a bad experience or been criticized. The worst that happens is they ask if you're comfortable talking on the phone. That's it, the worst, as bad as it gets. Horrifying, right? *Not.*

You want the job? You got this. Walk in there and find out what they need. Ask them! They have already spoken to ten people that week who sat there, too terrified to speak, and when they did open their mouths, all they did was answer short-vague questions about themselves. If you're still trying to be a non-stutterer and fit in with everyone else, then go for it. That's your comfort zone and what you should do. But if you want to get a job and further your career, *stand up and stand out*. Stutter on the first word of the first sentence. Get it out of the way and move on.

How you perceive your stutter is how others will perceive it. Change that self-perception and everything in your life will change. People see you as you see yourself. Seems crazy, and it's a difficult concept to fully grasp, but crazy or not it's true. Your body language says more about you than your words do. You can lie and your body will show it. You can fake confidence and your body will show it. Especially with women. Woman read body language five times better than men do. Don't even bother hiding anymore. It makes you feel awful and look oddly manipulative.

I spent most of my life as covert stutterer. That means I'm a walking Thesaurus of alternative words, which means I never mean exactly what I say or say exactly what I mean. It means I pretended not to stutter in the face of someone who obviously could see I stuttered. The awkwardness of that scenario creates anxiety and gives me shivers. I'm sure that others would have appreciated me just stuttering rather than insulting their intelligence with my brazen, ineffective con. I would act so weird, replace words in sentences that didn't exactly fit in them and hold a rigid-fake manikin smile the whole time. I was fake, inauthentic, and wasn't hiding anything. I felt fake because I *was* fake. I felt like I was lying every time I spoke, and it damaged me mentally. People seemed more exhausted than I did after conversations. It's as though they became lifeless and had no interest in me at all. I used to think it was because of the stutter but in reality it was like listening to someone tell a story for ten minutes that you knew was total bullshit. It's uncomfortable and drains people's energy, not to mention your own. If you do that, you really need to break that habit. It is severely unhealthy for yourself and your relationships.

Okay, so if you stutter you *are* different. Accept that. But isn't *everyone* different? If you pretend you don't stutter, if you struggle to be like everyone else, you'll be coming off as weird and you'll just make everyone around you feel weird too. Just admit it. Never put yourself down, but admit it to the person you're talking to. "I can't talk for shit today" is always a good opener. And you know what they'll do? Not a damned thing other than smile and appreciate you for breaking the tension.

There was a six-month period when I compulsively read relationship books. Every day. Seriously, like one or two a week for six full months. I was already in a relationship, but it was falling apart, and I wasn't quite sure why.

I knew that no book was going to repair that doomed relationship, but I realized I needed a much better understanding of the "operational" differences between men and women. The fact was that I'd become accustomed to treating every woman I met like a guy friend whom I'd had sex with. I began to understand that it might be attractive or "interesting" at first to be perceived as goofy or aloof or somewhat unattainable, but beyond the initial few weeks of a relationship, a woman needs to experience something deeper. As I kept reading dating books, pick-up artist books, new age books, Christian books, biology books, philosophy books, and psychology books, what intrigued me most and sent me on another journey was the issue of body language.

    This is where you can change your game. Your body says what you're thinking before you speak your thoughts aloud. It's completely subconscious and you can't prevent it. That means you're going to have to do some work on yourself, but it's worth it. If you are comfortable with your stutter, everyone you speak to will be comfortable with your stutter. If you freak out because you stutter, everyone else will freak out because you stutter.

    Your stutter creates a half-second of confusion in the minds of others and beyond that, they follow your lead. Besides, a half-second isn't exactly noticeable to most of the world. If you feel sorry for yourself, so will they. If you laugh at yourself, so will they. The fact is, If you think your stutter is a badass scar, so will they. People in the adult world are, overall awesomely tolerant of all sorts of things. Maybe because everyone is so damned preoccupied with their own crap, but trust me on this: No one is on a stutterers witch hunt and no one is hoping they can ruin someone's day. There are those rare individuals who are serious, full-time assholes, but you'd have to be living under a the spell of voodoo curse to encounter more than a small handful throughout your life.

Change the way *you* perceive your stutter, and I promise you it will change your life. If you can put this book down and remember one thing, please remember this. The way you see your stutter is how everyone else sees your stutter. Also keep in mind that there is not a sign on your forehead broadcasting the fact that you stutter.

Your stutter might catch people off guard...for about a second. They're not repulsed or inconvenienced or horrified or stunned into silence. They're simply caught off guard...for about a second. If someone walked up to you and stuttered you would be caught off guard too. When that guy turned around with a red ball in his eye socket I was like WTF. Then I saw the globe and anchor and he grinned and in a split a second my mind went from WTF to *thank you for your service, Hero.*

We stutterers are so self-conscious (ego centric?) that we're experts at projecting our negative bullshit onto others. If you walk into a room looking like someone just stole your bike, people are going to interpret everything you say and how you say it as that of someone who just had his bike stolen. If that's what you're looking for, if pity turns your crank and you want to die broke and lonely and begging for charity, then knock yourself out. It's your life. If you walk into a room like you're glad you're alive and everything is gonna be alright, then your stutter will be a sound for sore ears. People are tired of hearing about other people's problems. I know I am, and I'll bet you are too.

If you stutter, you are going to generate attention from anyone within earshot no matter how hard you try not to. It's just a fact you have to accept, but it's your choice what kind of attention it is. Are you having trouble finding someone to date? Observe yourself, what is your demeanor like? When a hot prospect sees you are you subconsciously telling them *Kick your shoes off and kiss me, Sexy?* Or are you subconsciously communicating *I'm special, would you please waste a year having pity sex with me and trying to fulfill my list of never-ending emotional needs?*

I am not being dramatic. People see this shit.

Do whatever you have to do to feel better. First step, get off your ass. Going for a walk will do this. Anything you do that moves your body will help. The more intense it is the better you'll feel. Walking will lift your spirits. Weight training, hiking, HIIT, yoga, martial arts—anything that demands effort and energy—will change your universe. Look outside. The guy 50 pounds overweight sitting on his porch smoking is not happy. You can feel his shitty outlook on life from across the street. The neighbor with the kayak and bikes on the roof of his Subaru?

He's probably a yuppie, but he's a happy yuppie with a lot more friends and who probably makes more money than you and the fat guy who smokes combined.

    When I'm feeling down, I walk a few miles with 90's baby-making music blasting from my headphones and singing horribly to the moon. Sometimes people cross the street and join in and they don't sing any better than I do. It's nutty, but it can be fun. My point is this: cheer the fuck up. Your stutter is what it is and you're making a much bigger deal about it than you have to . . . and that's not good for anybody.

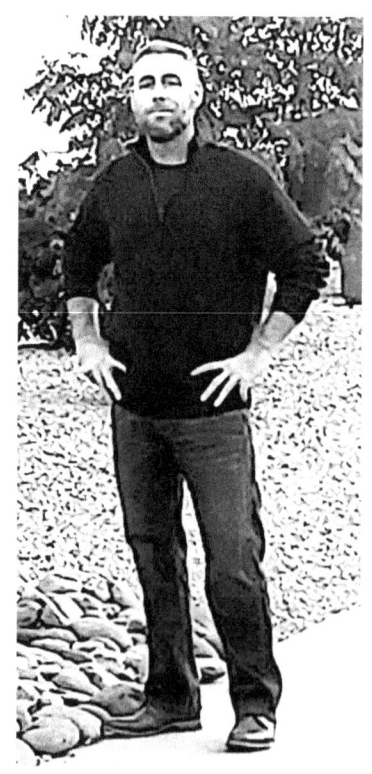

5.
Selling It

Doubt not, O Poet, but persist.
Say 'it is in me, and shall out.'
~Ralph Waldo Emerson

I love sales. A signed home improvement or remodeling contract feels so good in my hands it's like a natural high. It feels good because I do things the right way. I never lie to people or sell them anything they don't need. I ask them straight away. "What is it that you're looking for? Tell me what you want and I'll make it happen." I don't sell things to people, I serve people. They've worked hard for their home and probably saved up a long time to improve it. I treat every customer like I would treat my mom if she was sitting in that chair. Conventional sales techniques may work for people who don't stutter but they don't work for me.

I tell folks right off the bat that I am not a very good salesman. It breaks the ice, and they usually laugh and all the tension leaves the room. I want to know what their vision is and I will do anything I can to make it happen within their budget. I don't upsell, pressure or convince. I stutter, inform, and listen. I'm damn good at sales, I can't really explain why or how but I can explain how it feels. If I find myself feeling like I'm covert about my stuttering or if I find myself feeling slimy or inauthentic, it doesn't go well. If I feel like there's another person talking through me, I stop. I back away from the conversation mentally and imagine what I would feel like if this person was talking to my mom with his hand in her purse. I snap back to reality, act like myself and continue. That's it. We're all selling something, whether it's a product or services. We sell ourselves in job interviews, don't we? Be yourself and knowledgeable about your product, or your service, or...yourself.

    Salesman connect people to what they need. It would be really hard to buy anything without salesmen. What I'm saying is that as a stutterer, a sales pitch is useless and upselling is too exhausting. Talking is tiring, especially when you need to put in a little more effort to be fluent. It's okay to stutter during a meeting, but it's common sense that you need to make your point a little quicker than you would in a casual conversation.

    A stutterer can do anything they want for a living within reason. I'm not gonna tell you the world is your oyster and you deserve it because you merely exist. I'm saying that if you put the work in, educate yourself, master your craft, become comfortable in your own skin, and stop feeling sorry for yourself, there's a nice life waiting for you out there. You can use your innate and fine-tuned situational awareness and those work-around problem solving skills you began developing on the playground as a kid to make your own success story.

Tough Love

6. Addict

It does not matter how slowly you go along
as long as you do not stop.
~Confucius

I battled a drinking problem for ten years. It started innocently enough, I suppose. I discovered that a drink— or a couple or three or four drinks—gave me a nice little boost in confidence. Kinda took the edge off, y'know? I still stuttered when I drank but after a couple of shots or a six-pack, I basically didn't give two shits whether I stuttered or not. When I was drunk I was the guy I wished I could be sober. I had fun, got laid and made a million friends.

It was great . . . until it stopped working. The six-packs eventually didn't help all that much. But I fixed that little problem by making friends with my new compadre, Señor Bacardi. What a guy. Of course, I eventually had to drink the whole damned bottle of rum to feel the same way. Welcome to the world of spinning rooms and projectile puking.

Since the booze wasn't working as advertised, I starting taking pills with it. *Whoa.* That worked like a charm. I was back! Two rum and cokes and few valiums later I was the life of the party, the alpha male in the room, no fucks given!

Then . . . it somehow changed. It all stopped working completely and I was now chemically dependent, a full-fledged addict.

The only problem with being addicted to booze and pills is that when I was high, I couldn't control myself. I stopped being fun whether stoned, drunk, or agonizingly sober. I didn't drink socially. That's for lightweights. I drank every day. I verbally abused loved ones, became violent at times, and pushed away most of my friends. My family suffered, my career suffered, and I sure as hell suffered. It was seriously no fun, no matter how you look at it. I spiraled downhill mentally, physically, emotionally, economically. The alpha male was going limp in all respects.

By the time I finally came to my senses and got off the booze and pills, I suddenly discovered that I had to deal with the depression. Truth be told—and if you're not telling the truth you might as well shut the F up in my book—I missed alcohol; it had been my best friend for a long time, my wingman, my liquid courage. It saw me through many breakups and lonely nights. It let me drop the baggage I carried and have what felt like fun. It cheered me up when I was sad and celebrated with me when I was happy. That's what friends are for, right? The problem with alcohol, however, is that it's the kind of friend who easily reaches a hand into your pocket and steals the real you along with all your credit cards.

It was hard to do, but I managed to get my head straight and shake the booze off my back. Today, I can have two drinks—hey, nobody said I don't still enjoy a cocktail now and then—and call it quits. My fiancée knows she can trust me not to come home breaking shit and throwing up, and I know I can trust myself because I know—and truly believe—that I'm better than that.

Today, I can't say with anything approaching honesty that I drank excessively because I stuttered. That's a lame cop-out for anything. I gave myself a drinking problem for the same reasons any other addict does. I just blamed my stutter because that way I could get away with it. I had what I believed was a freakin' good reason for being completely out of control. When your fiancée says *I think your drinking is getting out of control* you can just pull out the handy ol' stutter card. "You don't understand how hard it is to be me! You can't judge me cause you don't stutter!" I knew my lines by heart.

If you've ever said those words to anyone, I hope I just pissed you off. I hope that you hate me right now for blowing your cover because we both know that's all it is: a lame-ass excuse for not dealing with the real issue, which is *you*. If you're abusing any substance because you stutter, you're a liar. You're abusing that substance to numb something or run from something that you don't have the courage or knowledge to deal with.

Stuttering comes with baggage. I acknowledge that, for sure. However; we exaggerate the stutter. We make it the defining thing about us and therefore the cause of all our problems. We also think were special because of it and any small accomplishment we achieve should be exaggerated because, after all, we're always the underdog.

Well, I hope you're sitting down, because I'm calling bullshit on that. If you're that serious about stuttering being that much of an issue, then please keep it to yourself so that the kids growing up with a stutter right now don't look at us and follow that sad, narcissistic example. My wish for the young stutterers is for them to see that what makes them different is also something that makes them stronger. I'll be damned if I'm gonna tell a young man that stutters he can use his speech impediment to harm themselves and others. I did, and years later I still have a hard time forgiving myself for it. I caused a lot of pain to myself and others, thinking that my stutter was the perfect justification. For that, I'm more than sorry.

Don't get me wrong. I'm not some holy-roller goody-two-shoes who's against drugs or alcohol. It's just that if I had been a more responsible person and had loved myself a little more, it would never have become a problem. I had a drinking problem because I felt sorry for myself. I hurt inside and I didn't know how else to numb it or deal with it. I knew it; I just didn't know what to do, or how to numb the pain. This isn't some sort of moral trip. I wasn't a bad person. I was just a lost person.

I didn't read or watch anything on TV other than football. I had no idea that self-help existed. It wasn't until I started fantasizing about suicide that I picked up a book.

No More Mr. Nice Guy by Dr. Robert Glover isn't even about addition. But it spoke to me. It changed a small part of me . . . and then another and then another. I didn't know it at the time, but I was learning to watch my own thoughts. Thoughts have no power over you if you're watching them and I was able to free myself from addiction by freeing myself from a faulty subconscious program. I didn't drink or take pills because I stuttered. I drank and took pills because I hated myself. When I learned to validate myself, stand up for myself and get my needs met in non-manipulative ways, I still stuttered but I realized I didn't want to hurt myself anymore. When I started taking care of my body, my family, and my heart, I found my masculine center. I still stuttered but I was still a man, a whole person, and I felt good about myself.

I now wake up every morning aware of my flaws and knowing what I need to improve. Stuttering is not on the list because I know the better I get the better my speech gets. I also wake up knowing that change is only a few books away. I have power over myself and am a loving master. I still stutter; I really don't care if it ever goes away. It doesn't cause any of my problems. If anything, it gives me the insight and compassion to solve problems in a way that opens up opportunities and beautiful relationships with beautiful people.

7.
Worthless

The only time we waste is the time spent thinking we are alone.
~Mitch Albom

Sympathy is like box of cookies. It feels good when you're shoveling them into your mouth but afterwards you feel like a sluggish piece of shit. Sympathy is your nemesis. Sympathy fuels the ego and diminishes your self-esteem. The attention feels good, the kindness of others puts a cute little cartoon-covered Band-Aid on the boo-boo you got when those kids made fun of you in 4th grade.

See the problem? You're holding onto something that happened in the 4th grade just so you can have a cookie. You're training your mind to get a dopamine hit by acting like a child. I understand that it hurts inside. Really, I get it. It creeps up in me all the time. I would get my ass kicked in school, get suspended for fighting back, then get my ass kicked at home because I got suspended for getting my ass kicked in school. Kids would follow me around telling me to say something and punching me in the back of the head until I did. I'd try say something just to make them stop pounding on me, but I'd verbally block to the point of gagging with my mouth stuck open, and they'd roll on the ground laughing. I watched one kid nearly hyperventilate. The little prick had to go to the nurse's office because he couldn't stop laughing so hard he couldn't breathe. That's how funny my stuttering was, a million laughs.

Not a single teacher ever helped me out. The only adult to ever intervene was a janitor who stopped a kid from nearly killing me in the fourth grade. The asshole kid was beating me with a book so hard I started to black out. He made the kid stop and then walked away. I limped home and got a spanking because the teacher said I wasn't paying attention in class. She was right. I was too scared at school to concentrate on anything but my next escape route. My life at school was one shitty day followed by another shitty day. That was life at school until I learned to fight back, which only got me expelled. I couldn't win. You want fair? Forget about it.

By the end of middle school, I'd learned to control the verbal blocks a little bit. Not really control them, but anticipate them, stop them before they had a chance to rise up in my throat and choke the words before I could get them out.

Things slowly began to improve. I found a couple of friends and the girls started noticing me. I had zero confidence but learned how to fake it. I got a little taller, learned how to dress, and got myself some awesome homemade tattoos. It was all a disguise designed to ingratiate myself with the crowd I hung out with. Dealing with bullies was no longer the issue; I could fight the best of them and, frankly, rather enjoyed it. So, by the 8th Grade, my act was working pretty well.

One day, I was at a "friends" house with six other boys, each doing his best to be a little hoodlum. They thought it was funny to make me say the word "ice" because I would completely block on the leading vowel sounds. My mouth would get stuck open as my throat strangled any sound attempting to come out. My eyes would roll to the back of my head. I was actually unable to see, almost blind for ten seconds. These guys wouldn't stop taunting me; for some reason they needed to laugh at me for the next hour. If I tried to go, I was afraid I'd get jumped and pounded. In that circle of punks, everyone had their turn "in the box," but no one else ever seemed to have as many turns as I did. It was all about enforcing a pecking order among the group, and I didn't have the social intelligence to maneuver through the situation very effectively. So I was destined to stutter for their entertainment or be forced to duke it out with some fool on a regular basis.

On this particular day, I gave in and tried to say "ice" just to keep the peace and stop the taunting. I tried not to block, but I did. My mouth got stuck open, my eyes rolled back, and when I opened them and could see again, one of these kids was standing in front of me, mimicking putting his dick in my mouth. The ultimate insult for a pre-teen boy.

Any other day, I would've taken a swing at the joker. But I didn't stand up for myself or fight. I just gave up inside, realizing I was only with this group to serve as a subject of their entertainment. That's all I was for these kids, a freak show. I existed for no other reason than to feed the sadistic needs of others.

I died inside that day. I started to cut myself and tried to break my knuckles on walls. The pain actually felt good because it made me feel *something*. I'd spend all night huffing spray paint from a paper bag and fantasizing about torturing people who made fun of me. I was dead inside, but beyond the numbing pain, deeper inside, I still had hope. I had my sister who always protected me. I acted tough and busted a few knuckles hitting those walls, but my sister was truly fearless. She loved me so much that I honestly believe that's why I'm still here. If I had killed myself, as I often thought I should, it would have destroyed her and I knew I could never do that.

When I was 15, I was a lookout while two of my friends burglarized a house. They stole a bunch of booze and cigarettes and then we binged on the contraband goodies. I blacked out drunk, completely passed out, and woke up in a pool of my own vomit as the sun was coming up; the start of another lovely day.

You'd think that would have been a lesson, but just before I blacked out, I remember feeling truly happy. I was happy because even though I stuttered, I didn't block when speaking. My friends were amazed by it and so was I. It was the first time I had been happy in so long. Genius that I was, I put 2 and 2 together. The solution to my speech problem was obvious, so I began to drink whatever I could find. A six-pack of beer, a couple of shots—or more—of tequila, and I was finally free to be the real me. People no longer made fun of me as long as I was half in the bag.

A little while later, I met my daughter's mom. I was the bad boy and she liked bad boys. Two years later my daughter was born, and—trying to be Mr. Responsible—I stopped drinking for two solid years. That baby—my beautiful daughter—was my salvation. I now had a purpose, a mission. I dropped out of continuation school, worked any job I could get to support our little family, and earned my G.E.D.

At 19, my stutter was less severe but my mental state had become awash in self-pity. I was doing well on the outside, but inside I was empty. I was still the stuttering kid living in terror of his next beat-down and everything about me was false, as though every minute of every day was a stage play.

It didn't take long for that marriage to fall apart. It was no one's fault; we were just kids. What did we know about marriage? Of course, I blamed the stutter, crying and cursing at God for this handicap. I was a lousy husband, not paying any attention to my young wife unless it was about sex. I'd hide out all night in the garage rebuilding cars and purposely worked the night shift for six months just so I didn't have to hear her complain about me not spending time with her. But I was avoiding everything, including her. I never admitted the reason or explained my behavior. But I knew it was the stutter. It was always the stutter.

My stutter caused constant pain. The stress and psychological effects built upon one another like layers of sediment throughout my childhood and haunted me right into adulthood. I had come to believe I was a worthless piece of shit because I stuttered. The only thing I had going for me was that I could make money with my hands and I wasn't the worst-looking guy in town.

After the inevitable divorce, I lived in my first bachelor pad with my daughter; we have some pretty good memories from that time and place. I made just enough to pay the bills, but all we really needed was each other. Of course, I did everything I could to hide my stutter from her. I was scared she would reject me or even start stuttering herself. I never spoke around her friends out of fear they'd tease her about my troubled speech. They came to believe that I was a great father because I was such a good listener. Her fluent voice was the only good thing in my world, and I cherished it. She's 24 now, and I marvel at and adore her fluency.

I went to work in my family's construction business. I worked my ass off and made good money. I loved construction, working with my hands, and creating something where nothing existed before. But I was still empty inside. I still needed something in my life with true meaning, something that would demonstrate my gifts and genuine potential. I needed to make my daughter proud of me. I needed to make myself proud of me, to do something that *matters*.

So I joined the Army Reserves and was quickly on my way to boot camp. Initially, I'd wanted to be a badass and shoot a cannon. I hoped to do something that made noise, had impact, changed the course of events. My recruiter had advised me to keep my stutter a secret if I wanted to get into artillery, but eventually an Army doctor picked up on it and disqualified me from working in combat arms. So I became a mechanic.

For a stutterer, daily life in the military can be a challenge because you're expected to speak quickly and fluently. I took a lot of shit from drill sergeants in what was clearly a serious version of the grown-up world. Things were different now.

Feeling sorry for oneself, offering excuses or explanations made no sense at all simply because nobody cared about my personal issues. I started to understand that and began to take it all with the dawning awareness that if I gave in to my frustrations, tried to explain things, hesitated, or faltered in my duty, I would become truly dead inside. I knew that if I crawled back home as a failure in the military I wouldn't be able to live with myself.

"What's your name, Private?" My drill sergeant yelled in his customary dulcet tones, slamming the hard brim of his cover into my forehead and spitting into my mouth at the top of his lungs.

"C-c-c-hapa, Drill Sergeant!"

"Are you fucking scared of me private?!"

"No, Drill Sergeant. I stutter, Drill Sergeant!"

Long pause, his eyes ripping my face apart. He stepped back, looked me up and down and said sternly "It's 'Private Chapa,' and you're not a worthless civilian anymore."

"Private Chapa, Sargent!" I yelled proudly, with everything inside of me, yelling fluently, my face flushing with sudden, unfamiliar pride.

"God-dammit Private, it's Drill Sargent! Drop! Push! Push! Push!"

He continued to yell at 1500 decibels, but it faded to white noise as I pushed and pushed and pushed. Tears fell out of my eyes, tears of joy. I'd never felt better. He didn't criticize me or make fun of me or belittle me. I was somewhere safe. I was in hell, but it felt more welcoming, more real, and more fulfilling than anywhere else I'd ever been.

I learned a lot in the Army. I became strong. My body could do anything and my mind was clear. I got teased a few times but it wasn't the same. It was friendly fire and everybody got their turn. Every day—even the occasional ribbing from the guys in my unit—was a test I was becoming strong enough to handle all of it. In the Army I had real friends. I wasn't there for their amusement. I was a soldier, we all wore the same gear, we overcame the same obstacles, and we were all equally "worthless."

I belonged.

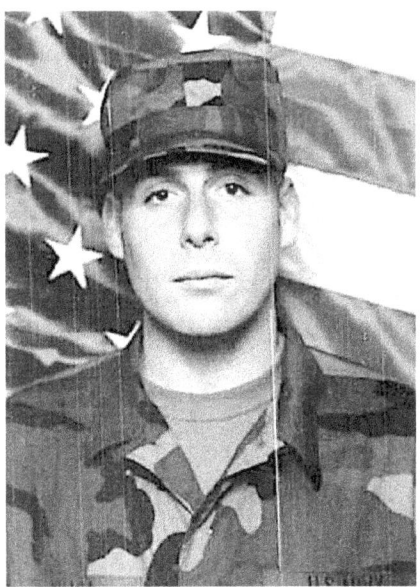

Tough Love

8.
Unfair

Life isn't fair. It never will be.
Go make life unfair to your advantages.
~Robert Kiyosaki

I could have—and probably *should* have—done things differently. Maybe not the early childhood stuff, but as a teenager I could have found better friends, made some better choices. I could have focused on my academic abilities or been more focused as an athlete. I'm not making excuses; I allowed a lot of things to happen because I was simply naïve, immature, or lacked the imagination to think of myself as more than I was defined as by others. We all know at least one lifelong, habitual, self-pitying martyr and we aren't all that eager to have long conversations or spend a lot of time with them. For a long time I was one of those martyrs. Feeling sorry for myself had become my default mind set.

As you grow up, you learn to take care of the wounded child inside you. In my reading and studies of masculinity, I did exercises speaking to my damaged inner child. It sounds corny at first, but when you feel like you are the protector of that little guy, you no longer draw energy from him; you advocate for his well-being and help him grow up. When that part of you grows up with your understanding and with your protection from harm, the rest of you grows up too.

Little Shane is still a brat who wants a cookie now and then, but now I toss him a protein bar and tell him to hit the books or the gym. He needs to get it together and move on because he's grown up now, life has worked out nicely, and things are better than just okay.

I feel a certain sense of gratitude and thankfulness when I remember that. Kids know when you're being strict for their own good and they love you for it later. They never like it at the time, but they always appreciate the benefits of the discipline that's been imposed upon them. I'm grateful that the US Army doesn't have room for self-pitying martyrs. The mission is pretty clear: Help the enemy to die for their country, but you get your buddies home. I despise pity now, from myself or others. I understand that it's no different than pills and booze. You never get enough, you become dependent on it, and it eventually destroys the person you're meant to be.

My drill sergeant had some sort of skin condition that was noticeable from his neck, around his face, to his head. He undoubtedly had experiences similar to mine—people staring at him or saying insensitive things—and had to get past them to be in the position he was. We all have our thing; we all have conditions, appearances, or histories we wish we could change. We've all got some level of faulty subconscious programming and a little kid crying with pain inside of us.

It's okay to cry when it hurts. It's not okay to cry for a cookie. I've learned to cry and I believe it's a powerful therapeutic tool if you allow it to be one. When my life becomes overwhelming and my emotions become so tangled to the point they become painful and impossible to deal with rationally, I just let it all out. Two minutes of tears and my mind is clear. My warrior archetype has vented his frustration at the situation, and I can then move on as a more productive and empathetic person. The frustrations of stuttering definitely builds up inside of you. Acknowledging that and letting it out can seriously make you feel better. You let go of the frustration. You let go of the tears. It's a great way to heal the pain, to diagnose the cause of the pain, and to rid yourself of it.

As humans in an ever-complex society we face a lot of anxiety. I'm working on my inner caveman now and he feeds off the tension when my anxiety gets ridiculously high. My stutter gets a lot its of energy from that anxiety. The more anxious I become, the harder it is to speak fluently. I've learned the science behind it and understand the biology of anxiety, but I'm all about hacks and getting to the bottom line to *fix it*. I don't give a shit what chemicals are making my brain go into fight or flight; it's nice information but ultimately useless.

I want to know the psychology and the causes and how to turn it all off. I want to lower the anxiety altogether, forever, and I've actually figured out how to do that. It's one of the harder things I've ever done, but it works and today I speak much more fluently because of my little hack. You're going to hate me throwing this out there because it's so generic. But stop shaking your head and please consider this because—I kid you not—it works.

It's a little thing called *confidence*.

Wait. Don't close the book, it's not what you think. Take a deep breath and hear me out. I'm not saying it's the cure-all for everything in life...but look around: Women love confidence, you make more money with confidence, games are won with confidence, presidents are elected with confidence. If my life proves anything, it proves that confidence is key!

Confidence really is the key—"the hack"—to a stutterer's success. But it's the hack that is so easily overlooked: we have more of it innately *because we stutter*. Remember when I said our default setting of fear is the same experienced by 90% of the general population at the mere thought of public speaking? That's our baseline. That's the absolute reality, the bottom line for us. You are stronger than you think. At the moment where fear arises—as you struggle to get the words out and get angrier at your inability to do so with every passing moment—you're putting yourself in the shoes of a fluent person and then you're judging yourself harshly because you're *not that fluent person.*

Think about it and you'll realize how irrational that is. Your speech is affected because you're afraid you're not going to be as good as everyone else...and 90% of them are just as scared as you are? That's like being afraid to play golf because everyone might discover you're not as good as Tiger Woods. Really?

Maybe it's time to get over yourself.

Maybe it's time to get out of some other person's shoes and get into your own. During your time on the planet, you've done everything that a fluent person has done, and you've done it with a stutter. You graduated high school with a stutter, you approached a girl or guy with a stutter, you got a job with a stutter . . . You've *lived* with a stutter. Your stutter has neither helped nor hindered you from accomplishing anything. Your stutter is just extra reps at the gym. It was a little harder and took a bit more energy, but your mind responded and you learned that it could do more than you ever thought.

We stutterers are different. No doubt about that. That simply means we have to look at things differently. To a fluent person confidence means believing you can do something. To a stutterer confidence means believing you can do something while worrying that someone will start a conversation with you or— God forbid—ask your name. (Why do stutterers always have a name they can't say? I think the first milestone in speech therapy should be to distinguish what letters the little guy blocks on and change his name accordingly. I mean seriously. Easy solution to an everyday problem. The system is corrupt!)

Your level of confidence--believing you can do something—is already there and it's actually stronger than you might think. You're like an elephant tied to a stick that is stuck in the ground.

The legendary Swiss psychiatrist Carl Jung proposed a psychological theory of development that symbolized the self approaching maturity as an elephant. When an elephant is born, its trainer tethers it to a small stick wedged into the ground so that it can't move. The elephant comes to believe that it can't go anywhere if it is tied to the stick. Years later, when the elephant is full-grown and obviously strong enough to rip a phone pole out of the ground, the trainer can still tether it to the same little stick and the elephant will still believe it can't go anywhere. It's obvious a full grown elephant can go wherever it wants, but it's been *programmed* into believing it can't so it sits on its ass and waits for the trainer to untie him. That's all therapy is, a process of changing your belief system.

This is all self-development stuff, and that's all it takes to have the confidence to succeed: a change in your belief system. It's understanding that at one time you couldn't pull the stick out of the ground but you're bigger and smarter now, so you can. If you're an adult, you *must*. It's called growing up and taking responsibility for yourself, for who you are and what you can accomplish.

You can't get that job because you stutter? Maybe you couldn't when you were younger because your only qualifications were a high school diploma and a soccer participation trophy, but if your resumé is in anyway close to the job description you want, you can *get that job*. Unless there's a sign on the door that says "No stutterers allowed!" the only one discriminating against anyone is you. You're discriminating against yourself, which simply doesn't make any sense.

You've lifted all the weights everyone else has; you've just done a few more reps because you've been tied to a bigger stick. I don't care how big that stick is. Pull the damned thing out of the ground. Now you're an elephant with a big stick. Big sticks swing harder and don't break as easy. You're not as poorly equipped for success, life, and love as you thought you were.

Confidence is not about convincing yourself you can do something, its letting go of the belief that you can't.

My first day in the Army I did 13 pushups. After nine weeks of basic training I did 100. It's impossible to increase your strength by 900% in nine weeks. The fact is, I could already do 100 pushups on that first day. I just didn't believe I could, so I couldn't. I just needed proper motivation.

In Basic Training, touching a drill sergeant's hat is punishable by death. I mean it, you might die. At the very least, you'd roll around in the mud all night purely for his entertainment. That first week, I couldn't hold myself in the pushup position for longer than a few minutes. My arms would shake and I would collapse onto my chest. But when a drill sergeant puts his hat underneath you and says "I dare you," your arms miraculously get strength you never dreamed of and you can hover above that hat, suspended on a cloud of I-don't-wanna-die for a solid hour. It's all about your perspective and having the proper motivation. No, I really didn't think he would kill me, not literally. But there was no doubt he'd think I was a punk and not good enough to be a soldier in his Army.

What's your drill sergeant hat? What truly motivates you? What do you need to get past your mental blocks? My motivation is my family. They've seen me fail and it hurts. It's the worst pain I've ever felt. Pain like that can kill you, so I know I won't do it again. I will not fail in front of my kids again. *Because I stutter* is not an acceptable explanation for why you're not supporting your partner, being involved in your kids' lives or why you're fucking up yours. You can't change your childhood. You just have to reframe it as extra reps or realize you can rip that stick out of the ground and go wherever you want with it.

Here's the secret to this whole stuttering "thing": *There is no secret. It's all hard work.*

Now you know.

So now you need to do the hard work. If you're needy, learn to validate yourself. If you're shy, stop describing yourself that way and get over yourself. If you stutter, go talk to as many people as you can (serious immersion therapy!) and soon enough you'll realize that nobody but you actually gives a shit about your stutter. Instead of wringing your hands over yourself (stutterers are notorious perfectionists and narcissists), focus on what you want to change about yourself and start reading about it. The more you read, the more you'll know. The more you know...the more you'll be able to accomplish.

~ ~ ~

A while back, I was scrolling through a Facebook group for stutterers that my friend joined and then invited me to join as well. First damn page…"I'm 43, I'll never find love or a job. It's so unfair."

Seriously? It's so unfair? It's unfair that you had a rough childhood but at 43 it's your fault if your resume is subpar and you still judge other people so harshly that you can't approach them? Give me a break. Whoever wrote that fits the paradigm of the "poor me, I stutter" self-defeated narcissist who is his own worst enemy.

Look, I understand the need for children to be validated and told repeatedly how awesome they are (even when they're just an average kid). What really bothered me about that Facebook page is that there are kids on it, being exposed to all this self-defeating stuff. Is this how kids who stutter should feel about themselves? Is this what kids should be exposed to when they're trying to get through high school with a stutter? Shame on the dipwads who post that stuff.

I'm not intentionally trying to hurt anybody's feelings here, but everything I'm telling you here is from my own personal experience and pain as a "stuttering survivor." It took me 30 years to stop blaming my stutter, to stop being a loser. That was the mindset that cost me everything I worked for, twice. I wasn't a loser because I was a 30 something stutterer; I was a loser because my perspective of reality was that of a ten-year-old stutterer.

I want to be a part of the stuttering community, but I don't want be a part of one filled with losers who have already given up. If you're a hard-charging winner who's willing to do the hard work of dealing with the hand we've been dealt, if you're a person who puts a value in yourself far beyond the "stick in the ground" that can never define who you really are or limit what you're capable of, then I want to be in *your* group.

9.
Other People

The unhappiest people in the world are those who care most about what other people think.
~Mother Theresa

Have you noticed something?

When you stutter, people notice.

Other people. Everyone in line behind you, everyone at the dinner table, waiters, people at the table across the room... anyone within hearing distance of your voice.

It's weird. You can feel eyes move in your direction. You can feel the heat of attention shifting toward your every utterance. Blood rushes to your face, your heart speeds up, your breath shallows and your brain goes into fight-or-flight mode. You either want to disappear or turn around like "What? You never heard someone say please with three p's before? What's wrong with *you?*"

In the process of writing this, I asked a lot of people a lot of questions. I really wanted to know how they reacted to hearing a stutter. The answers were honest; the data compounded a list of reactions and thoughts that were so predictable and clichéd that I actually had to get creative to even describe it all.

Stuttering? Incredibly, no one cared. The most dramatic reaction I heard was sympathy for the stutterer. Most everyone reported that they knew someone who stuttered, so my questions reminded them of that person.

As I sat at my desk analyzing these reactions I realized how mind-blowing they actually were. I asked ex-girlfriends what they thought the first time I spoke to them. The consensus was something like *I was more worried about you being a player and I didn't really think about it.*

I asked coworkers and friends what they thought when they first met me. The majority reactions were things like *I was hoping I wasn't being rude in any way when you were talking. After a day I kinda didn't notice it anymore.*

These answers amazed me because so much of stutterers' anxiety and fear of stuttering is based upon *the fear and anxiety of stuttering*. How's that for a vicious circle?

Fear and anxiety of what? If nobody cares that you, I, we stutter, what the hell are we so uptight about? I've already described the stupid childhood stuff, and I've already gotten resolved all of that in my own life, yet I still feel this anxiety running through so many personal situations.

I dug deeper, analyzed the situations. I tried speaking louder to cashiers and waited for reactions from those in the line behind me. I walked up and introduced myself to the new guys at work. I pulled my truck over at an intersection and asked someone sitting at a crowded bus stop for directions.

I took chances, risked embarrassment, and still I couldn't get a single reaction from anybody that was inconsistent with my previous assessments. Not one person cared if I stuttered or reacted when I did. I tried to get reactions; I blocked harder than a rookie tight end in the 3rd week of preseason. I was tempted to hit on a lady at the bookstore to see how that went but I didn't think my fiancée would approve of my exhaustive research, even for the sake of science.

If you hang out on online stuttering forums, 99% of the discussions consist of horror stories and tales of emotional devastation. In my adult life, I have yet to experience this. I'm 5'8" and 170lbs. I walk around with a goofy smile and I'm usually consciously polite. I am in no way intimidating to others, so it can't be that. At work I talk to at least 10 people I've never met every day. I'm a small town guy and often start conversations standing in line among total strangers. I go to bars and coffee shops with my friends, talk to all my neighbors, and make the same number of phone calls a fluent person does in their day-to-day life. Once in a while someone hangs up the phone because I take too long to say something, which can be a little annoying. But when I call back and they realize I stutter, it quickly becomes apparent that—like every other example I've noted in this chapter—they don't seem to really give a shit.

I was missing something. The common denominator: Me. I used to have all kinds of stories about cashiers being rude to me or customers not having time to listen to me, and I used all of it as a rationale for my drinking. I was reacting to women mistreating me, police harassing me, and all the subtle discrimination I faced in the business world. That all infuriated me...and so I drank. I sat in my truck and cried about it and got mad at my fiancée because she didn't understand the suffering I endured every day.

That was my story, and I stuck to it.

But here's the truth of the matter: None of that actually fucking happened. At the time I believed it did. At the time it was a 100% accurate version of my daily experience.

But it never happened.

It was all my own twisted perception of reality. Life was hard and I needed a reason for all my difficulties other than the reality of my own abysmal immaturity and self-pity. I was going through a hard time in life because the world was against me, so I had to validate that perception somehow. Whenever someone was rude to me or didn't agree with me, my perspective—my internal reaction—was actually my perspective of myself. I was perfect, I was the victim (dare I say "martyr"?) and the only thing wrong with me was my speech. I became an expert at projecting my unseen self-rejection onto others and soliciting their negative responses. Those negative responses were actually a reflection of my shitty attitude and had nothing to do with my speech. Arguments, disagreements, and rejections were, in fact, responses to my manipulative need for constant validation, and had nothing to do with my speech. Being combative, self-righteous, verbally aggressive, and argumentative is what turned people off. Not the stutter.

When I finally began working on myself—not my stutter, myself—my self-image changed. As my self-image slowly evolved, what I projected onto others changed as well. As my projections, behavior, and tone changed, everyone else seem to change. *Maybe no one is making fun of you. Maybe you're making fun of yourself?* When I began to realize this, I came to understand that this really is a beautiful life full of good people. Turning your back on that truth just so you can feed some deep-seated need to feel special can really fuck your life up.

If this is actually happening to you, if you are being verbally or mentally abused, you are in a bad situation. You are not around normal or mentally stable people and you need serious help to get out of that situation. I'm not kidding. What you're facing is not okay and you need help. I still know those boys who tortured me as a child; today they're adult men who would never act like that or allow their children to. The majority of people do change and grow up. A small percentage don't, and if you choose to associate with those, then you're only bringing the pain of those relationships onto yourself.

Look, I'm not trying to bring anyone down. I'm merely trying to drop the curtains on a bad play. This is a book about stuttering, and I suppose I could name all the famous people throughout history up to the present moment who have stuttered and tell you that at one time they couldn't say hard consonants either. While that may be accurate, it's become something of a cliché, like enumerating all the famous people who suffer from dyslexia.

It's simply beside the point to report that there are stutterers somewhere near the top of every profession who surely didn't get there by obsessing over their speech impediment. They did what they could to speak as fluently as they could but focused on achieving success and not on their speech challenges. The stuttering CEO doesn't wake up thinking about 4th grade bullies. She/he wakes up thinking about staffing, supply chains, cost management, and improving revenues. The stuttering lawyer doesn't go to bed and read a book about how to stop stuttering. He's reading about how to win the next case, start his own practice, or become a law firm partner.

The more you concentrate on your career, your health, and building relationships, the less you stutter. If I told you not to think about a pink elephant, you will think about a pink elephant.

You can't turn it off; you can only make the pink elephant fade away by thinking about something else.

The more you obsess over your stutter, the more you *will* stutter. Let it fade away and go live your life. Find your purpose and follow it. What would you do with your life if you didn't stutter? Be honest with yourself: if you spoke with total fluency, what would change? How would you be different? What job could you have that you don't think you can have because you stutter? What dream do you have that you can't fulfill because you stutter?

Of course, there are individual situations and limitations. Some stutter so severely that speaking at all is nearly impossible. If that's the case then what is there to lose? If you cannot speak at all but you spent every waking hour improving yourself in every other way, who's to say your speech wouldn't follow suit? That's exactly what worked for me. I used to stutter on every word I said. Once I stopped obsessing over it and began working on other aspects of my life and learned the value of self-help, my stuttering pattern changed. Today, I typically only block on the first word, and in casual conversation I don't block at all.

Speech therapy might not help you (I never did it as an adult), so you'll need to focus on the rest of "you," to explore other aspects of your being. If you become 100% fluent but you're still 100% overweight, 100% broke, and 100% mentally fucked up, what difference will speech fluency make in your life?

You would fluently be upset that you were unhealthy, broke and depressed.

I want you to know that I love you and I understand the insanity that stuttering can cause and the havoc it can wreak on your life. We have to be honest with ourselves and with our stuttering: there is no cure. I've researched them all, and I doubt if there will be a cure any time soon. Waiting for the magic pill that's going to change your life is like refusing to look for a job because you're sure that you're going to win the lottery any day now. That's just not going to happen, okay? (If it does, let me know and I'll gladly refund the entire price of this book.)

The only proven strategy to live a good life as a stutterer is to do just that: **live a good life as a stutterer**.

10.
Own It

What makes you different or weird,
that's your strength.
~Meryl Streep

Being different is good . . . if you own it.
My fiancée and I went to a posh brunch for our anniversary yesterday. I laughed inside, studying the menu and remembering how things were just a few years ago and how I used certain strategies to just get through the day.

Early in our relationship, I would get a rhythm going with my foot till I could spit out what I wanted off the menu, then excuse myself to the men's room, telling her to order for me if the waiter came back. It was no different than going to the little boys room right before it was my turn to read in front of the class. I was too ashamed to stutter in front of her or deal with the awkwardness of stuttering to the waiter while she sat there stirring her coffee far longer than it takes to mix cream into it. I was certain that my stuttering would ruin the ambiance of date night with eyes and giggles directed at us from other tables. I saw my disfluent speech as a freak show and perceived any type of attention or curiosity as proof.

But the point came when I couldn't keep heading to the restroom every time we went to dinner, and I confessed my strategy to her. The solution seemed simple enough: she started ordering for me voluntarily. She knew how insecure I was about my stutter and, like most people who love someone who stutters, she was happy to help me out as much as she could.

I always acted like it wasn't a big deal, but in reality it was. I often felt like her child. She's a natural caretaker and I think a part of her liked speaking for me, but it was not healthy for me or for our relationship. I realized that the convenience of the arrangement was detrimental to the polarity of our relationship.

There is an ebb and flow that manifest itself between lovers. This energy fluctuates, and it can dissipate desire or generate greater romance. A stutter does not interfere with this energy, but the relationship a stutterer has with his stutter can fuel it or completely smother it.

My fiancée used to make phone calls for me as well. She'd get upset because they didn't understand my affliction and she kicked ass for me on the phone just like my mom did when I was a kid and she was fighting with the school on my behalf. My fiancée is an awesome mom. My mom is an awesome mom. But my fiancée is not my mom and acting like she is doesn't do much in the way of building a healthy romantic relationship.

A few years ago we were out for dinner with her son who had gotten himself into trouble at school. We were only eating out because we were both too tired to cook at home. She'd had a hard day at work and we were bickering. The waiter approached the table as the discussion turned to what the kid wanted for dinner, which was the usual junk food. Already exhausted, she compromised with him and turned her attention to me with an expression on her face that rocked my masculinity to the core. It was the same expression she'd had while arguing with her boy about ordering vegetables instead of fries. Her eyes challenged me to tell her what I wanted for dinner, expecting me to point to something on the menu.

I'll never forget that moment. I felt completely emasculated as a wave of frustration, resignation, and disappointment came over me. "Go ahead," I said.

Her tired eyes said it all: *just point at something already, I'm hungry*. It seemed like time slowed down, but it was just my thoughts in hyper-speed. I was afraid to stutter in front of the waiter. I was afraid to stutter in front of her. I was afraid that people in the nearby booths would turn and look at us with curious pity.

When you're full of yourself, you feel that everybody is paying attention to you and when you pity yourself, you *hope* they are. At that moment, I had both that feeling and that hope. I wanted her to be a partner in that moment, not a parent. She needed a lover who was decisive and able to express his needs clearly and fluently. This may seem like I'm making a big deal over ordering a cheeseburger, but it actually was. I ordered my food. Stuttered, blocked, and finally got it out, unable to breathe, the wind knocked out of me, wanting to gulp for more air. The waiter didn't even react. He didn't seem to care, and no one near us exploded in laughter as she fixed me in her gaze the whole time. I couldn't feel my own jaw, numb with stress, but I could feel her vibration change as she realized things would be different from then on.

It was difficult at first, but I knew then that I could never go back to an arrangement where she would be ordering dinner while I escaped to the men's room. Ever since then, I order my own food and make my own phone calls. I don't feel the need to compensate for my masculinity and she doesn't have to change roles from partner to parent between appetizers and the main course. It seems so petty to be so afraid of such mundane things, but as a stutterer such mundane things can be the source of genuine trauma. The trauma may only be a perception and have no basis in reality beyond the stutterer's but that's not the point. It takes courage to face it and deal with it.

If you hold a finger in front of your eye, you can hide the moon. If you put your fears in front of reality they can hide opportunity. When you experience trauma as a child, it's magnified, and as an adult it affects how you see yourself and the world.

As a child, I'd learned that if I stuttered, people would hit me. I'd also learned that women would baby me. I became anxious about stuttering in public simply because my subconscious sensed danger. I'd let my fiancée take care of things and protect me from my own perceived embarrassment because it feels good to be taken care of. It wasn't because I was weak or afraid of anyone. It was a mix of adrenaline and other hormonal responses being triggered by my brain, the same brain that moves my lungs and heart without me being consciously aware of the workings of my own autonomic nervous system. Once I became aware of this internal wiring, I learned how to control it. If you pay attention to your lungs you can control them. If you stop, they go back to autopilot and they continue to function without any conscious effort at all. The brain-body connection is truly an awesome autonomous system of chemical impulses, electric circuits, and motor functions. Things just work with or without our constant attention. Our responses to stimuli from the outside world are no different. My fiancée is scared of roller coasters because as a kid she almost fell out of one. Intellectually, she knows roller coasters are safe because she's taller now, but her emotional memories and psychological triggers stimulate her internal chemistry and she still trembles a bit when standing in that amusement park line.

We stutterers have often been physically abused, beaten up, or verbally humiliated when our speech falters. We get anxious when we need to speak because we haven't realized we're actually "taller" now. By adulthood, most stutterers are twice as fluent as we were as adolescents. But the old patterns, the programs imprinted on us from childhood, still remain. As I took the reins and began speaking for myself more and more, I stuttered less and less. My brain was able to rewrite the program it had created as a result of negative inputs, and my the dial on my anxiety meter began to move from from Extreme to Mild. I still get anxious before speaking, but there are times when I speak with total fluency without even realizing it. The minute I do notice it, of course, I begin to block and the stuttering returns like an obnoxious friend you can't quite shake.

11.
Growing into It

Who looks outside, dreams.
Who looks inside, awakes.
                              ~Carl Jung

Any stutterer would consider waking up one day without a stutter even better than winning the lottery. There's a catch though: there are several economic studies that show how most people who win the lottery declare bankruptcy within three years. Lottery winners become instant millionaires without really having a clue what it's like to be a millionaire.

Being a millionaire isn't really about the money at all; it's a mindset. Millionaires have problems the average wage-earner can't comprehend and experience stresses that can only be understood by other millionaires.

The same holds true for fluent speakers. They have perspectives and mindsets that a stutterer does not comprehend. If an everyday blue collar individual becomes a millionaire his bank account changes but his financial intelligence, subconscious programming and perspectives remain the same. To be successful as a millionaire you have to psychologically become a millionaire. Self-made millionaires are able to maintain their wealth because they grew psychologically as their financial footing evolved.

When I decided to speak for myself, I began reprogramming my subconscious. Because my subconscious now understands my determination to speak for myself, that self-pity is pointless, and that nothing horrible is going to happen, my speech has improved. I now understand that there may be a neurological synapse-glitch in my brain that causes me to stutter and that fighting my stutter or catering to only makes it a bigger problem than it needs to be. The physical stutter that I have today is so slight that most people wouldn't notice it. The explosions, ambushes, and ordnance of blocks and repetitions in my speech are merely sounds of the battle within.

Imagine yourself speaking fluently. Imagine standing tall with your chest out, chin up, and shoulders back. Imagine your throat completely relaxed and your lips moving only as words are spoken and released, not before. Imagine yourself smiling and laughing as you speak. If you can imagine it, it exists. If you can't imagine that fluency, it's only because you don't want to. If you don't want to, it's only because you're getting something out of it..

Maybe it's time to have a serious conversation with yourself and figure this out.

What do you have as a stutterer that you would lose if you suddenly became fluent? What if you woke up tomorrow completely fluent? If you won the speech lotto and could miraculously speak perfectly, what would change? You'd feel great, an overwhelming sense of freedom would flood over you, and the success following your eloquent pronunciation of words would fall into your lap from unicorn wings. Love, wealth and happiness would enrapture you in an ever-flowing gracious breeze of blessings!

Really? You think so? (If you do, let me tell you about this bridge I have for sale...)

The reality is that if you were suddenly fluent, life might get harder. Fluency, like money, doesn't make you who you are. It only magnifies it. You'd realize that people used to go out of their way to be polite to you. Some people felt sorry for you and didn't call you out when you were an asshole. You'd realize that you have no excuse to be less than your best and you'd eventually understand that everything you thought was the fault of the stutter is still there. You'll still be nervous at job interviews, introductions and at the prospect of approaching someone you're attracted to. You'd still be co-dependent, self-loathing and uninspired. The only difference would be you'd no longer have an excuse for any of your shortcomings. If a bill collector calls you can't avoid the conversation because you "can't talk." If you can't find a job, wouldn't be able to blame the phone interview or the oppressor on the other end. You also can't blame your mistakes as a partner or a parent on your inability to communicate effectively.

People who don't stutter have just as many problems as people who do. People often blame their failures on how they were raised or the neighborhood they grew up in. Everyone today is WebMD self-diagnosed OCD, ADHD and depressed. Everyone has a reason that they are not living up to their potential or disciplining themselves. Are you holding onto your stutter because it's such a convenient excuse to avoid those things that scare the shit out of you? If you blame any lack of achievement on your stutter, the answer is obvious...and your stutter is just one way to excuse your lack of success, your lack of determination, your lack of persistence, your failure. That's the very definition of "cop out." If fluency was all you needed to live the life of your dreams, every fluent person would be living the life of their dreams. Whether your dream is to become a fluent speaker or a millionaire, you have to own that dream. Your chances of one day waking up completely fluent are less than the odds of winning the lotto. You can't win the lottery if you don't buy a ticket, and you can't improve your speech without a healthy dose of discipline and hard work.

12.
The Card

The only thing standing between you and
your goal is the bullshit story you keep telling yourself.
~Jordan Belfort

I have friends who smoke medical marijuana for depression, and after smoking weed for 10-15 years, they're still depressed. I'm not for or against marijuana—I really don't understand how it qualifies as a political position—but I have to ask the question: If you take medicine every day for 10-15 years and you still have the condition that you take the medicine to treat, is it at all possible it's not working for you? Let me put it another way: Is it conceivable that your depression is still there *because you reward it by getting high every day*? I've had this conversation with my friends and the truth always reveals itself with a sly grin. They smoke weed *because they like it*. Depression is just their excuse to smoke weed.

The next question I ask is pretty obvious: Why don't you just smoke weed because *you like smoking weed*? Before the recent wave of cannabis legislation making it legal to sell grass on every street corner, the answer was always the same: "Well, if I'm depressed, I can get a medical card and buy it legally." (Now that marijuana is increasingly legal nationwide, I'll bet there are a lot of "mental health" marijuana "card" prescription-writers looking for another line of work.)

I think we all have a "card" of some type. A license to chill. I had a wallet full of them and still keep some hidden that I know I should toss in the trash. I have a *I can eat junk food because I have a physical job* "card," a *I don't have to master composition because I'm an abstract writer* "card" and of course I have everybody's favorite *I was raised that way* "card." These metaphorical "cards" hold the same power as a physical card. These cards allow you to do things and they allow you to avoid doing other things.

I didn't give up my stuttering card. Instead, I just let it expire. I still have it. I try to pull it out once in a while when I'm struggling in daily life, but it's not valid anymore and no one I know will accept it. I made the choice to live as I would if I didn't stutter and I do. If I don't make a business call I should have made, it's only because I was lazy, not because I couldn't talk. If I don't go for that awesome job or start that business, it's because I wasn't motivated to do so, not because I can't handle the conversations that might be involved.

My "card" simply doesn't work anymore because once I stopped self-medicating with self-pity, my stutter became less severe. Here's the reality: I wasn't doing any of it on purpose. I just wanted to be a better person. Stuttering or not, I wanted to like the guy I saw in the mirror. The more work I did on myself the less I needed an excuse not to actually *do the work*. I learned that it feels good to dig yourself out of the hole you were thrown into, to climb out of that hole victorious and to like the person looking back at you in the mirror.

Tough Love

13.
The Magic Pill

The secret to the Magic Pill is that
there is no Magic Pill.
~Deepak Chopra

We've all thought about it, hoped for it, imagined it, dreamed it: the secret elixir that scientists are working on day and night to treat an affliction affecting over 70 million people. That's a lot of people and whomever discovers and brands "Fluentix" is going to be an overnight billionaire. I can't wait to see the TV commercials!

Imagine driving home from the pharmacy with those little pills in a little brown bottle, gift-wrapped in a little white paper bag. You were going to take the pill in the parking lot, but you wanted to make it a special occasion so you wrap the passenger seat belt around it to keep it safe and carefully pull out onto the street. You're driving with one eye on the road and one eye on the bag. Your foot is shaking on the pedal. Your heart is pounding at cardio speeds. You breathe in deeply to calm yourself as you pull into your driveway. You're so excited you can't get the key in the door, so you sit on the porch, ankles spread, knees tight, pigeon-toed like a kid with a bag of Skittles who won't share and now you rip off the top of the bag. Your hands reach into the bag, ceremoniously retrieving the key to greatness from its 50% recycled treasure chest. Your mind is spinning in a vortex of metaphysical parallel realities and the possibilities awaiting you in The Realm of the Fluent. To hell with all the snide remarks and years of abuse you've suffered. You are the king and vengeance shall fall upon those who have found you unworthy. The shroud encasing the mystical capsule proclaims warnings, carved perfectly onto its surface by the scribes of Faraday's Law. This miracle is too powerful for those under 10 to handle and you roll your eyes at yourself as you struggle to release the childproof lid. Slowly you turn the lid opening the treasure chest containing all of your wildest dreams and allow the concoction of snake venom and roots from faraway lands to spill onto your anxious palm. This moment is yours. Your freedom awaits as you fearlessly consume the answer to your dreams without anything to wash them down. You close your eyes. A sense of calm fills you as you mentally take your seat at the table of those who didn't go to speech class for third period instead of art…where they got to practice calligraphy. You meditate.

      You envision the phoenix rising from the ashes into the air screaming vowels and hard consonants with ease as it flies into the sun. You feel it. The tightness in your jaw and throat dissipates into your aura and grounds itself under your feet. You speak but you speak to no one in particular. You speak only to speak as you fluently articulate all the words you have never said because you dodged them and replaced them with other, easier words.

It's time to share the blessings of the muse held captive in your constricted throat.

You call your family and friends together. Unbridled affection and pride emanate from those who adore you as they anticipate the bounty delivered by the gods of Speaking Mercy. Your friend asks, "Do you feel different?"

Your mind races to Jupiter and back, unable to define the feeling of your long-awaited healing. Your mind wanders into the cavern of double arches as you fearlessly order whatever you want at the drive-thru. You summon the courage to even dare call the cable company and have them upgrade your service because your Fantasy Football team had a great draft and you don't want to miss the blacked-out home games. The cashier at the coffee shop who writes hearts on your cups has no idea that tomorrow—before you go to work and ask for a raise because you're totally awesome now—you will ask her for her phone number!

Wake up, dude.

You're still gonna text her because you have her on a pedestal and some PUA ("pick up artist") douche on YouTube told you to wait three days. That's if you actually manage to get her number because she was attracted to the cute guy who stutters but wasn't too shy for small talk. Your boss is going to be offended that you think he evaluates your job performance by your speech and in three days all those people who celebrated with you won't care anymore for a very simple reason which you never even considered until it hit you right between the eyes: *they never did care.*

If you suddenly become fluent—if you actually find that "Fluentix" commercial, pick up the phone to dial that 1-800-STUTTER number and order your first bottle with Express Shipping—nothing will really change at all. Okay, so a few things will become more convenient. But that's it, my friend. The rest of your life is still *the rest of your life.*

Your stutter simply does not affect you as much as you think it does. If you could speak fluently, would you know exactly what to say in any situation? Would you have the confidence to ask someone out and call them that night just to get to know them better? Consider this: What if your stutter was the thing that people found most interesting about you? What if instead of humiliating, your stutter was humanizing. What if you made people feel free to be themselves and show their own shortcomings, foibles, and rough edges? What if your inability to articulate every word perfectly gave others the ability to articulate their feelings more clearly? What if they are so tired of having to fit in to an airbrushed notion of an perfectly unflawed social milieu that you are actually a breath of fresh air, a pleasant relief to be around? Just imagine...*what if?*

Tough Love

14.
Stand Up, Stand Out

In order to be irreplaceable
one must always be different.
~Coco Chanel

Imagine you're presenting a proposal to a client. They have you scheduled at 3:00 p.m. for a 30-minute appointment. You're dressed to impress, you've stopped at the barber's to get touched up and mentally prepared for any questions they might have. In the receptionist office, you tap your finger nervously on your laptop bag and breathe into your stomach to calm the butterflies. The motivational posters on the wall in glossy black frames keep your mind busy, lost in their clichéd rhetoric. The door to the conference room opens and your competition exits, dabbing the dew from his forehead. He nods as your eyes meet. The receptionist politely calls your name and you confidently rise. You enter the conference room, extend your hand to your prospective client and smile as you greet them. You can feel your throat tighten, but you've done this before and purposely stutter with "I-I-I appreciate you making the time to see me. I-I-I hope I can help you guys out."

They acknowledge your stutter with their eyes and thank you in return for coming in. You sit across from them, retrieve your notebook and ask, "What is your o-o-bjective on this project?"

They tell you what they are looking to accomplish and what services they need. You point out a logistical discrepancy they overlooked and they thank you for noticing it. The meeting goes well. They're clearly impressed by your knowledge in the field, and you shake hands, thanking them again for their time. As you leave the conference room, you come face-to-face with another subcontractor nervously tapping his foot waiting for his appointment. You wish the receptionist a great day and leave the office. You stuttered more than you wanted too but didn't block too much, and the conversation went as smoothly as you could have hoped for. It's Friday, you're off for the weekend and you're on the way to meet your buddy at the pub to watch the game.

A few hours later, you're sitting on a barstool across from your buddy at a small round table. The game is about to start and you decide to get a few beers before the bartender gets busy. You stutter over the loud ambient noise and blink hard. The bartender nods and retrieves two glasses from the chiller. You also caught the attention of a woman a few barstools away who's talking with another woman or two. You smile, she smiles, and you break eye contact to pay the bartender. It's a good football game on the TV monitors hanging above the bar. The woman you noticed is being noticed by other men nearby, but she obviously just wants to hang out with her girlfriends. Besides, a shouted conversation among other noisy bar patrons is not exactly supportive of your speech patterns.

As you leave the bar, you write your number on a napkin and slide it down the bar towards her. She graciously accepts it with a smile and you maneuver your way out of the pub and through the rear exit. She has a great night with her friends, politely excuses herself from a growing phalanx of potential suitors, and she leaves to go home to binge-watch her favorite TV series and shake off the work week.

You were one of eight subcontractors who pitched proposals to your prospective clients earlier that day. They have two weeks to turn in accepted proposals to their superintendent , so they tabled your proposal along with all the others and took off for the weekend.

Over the weekend they live their lives and spend time with their family and friends. Later that week they reconvene in the conference room to discuss the project that you bid on. By that time, they've forgotten 90 percent of everything that happened back on Friday in those meetings with you and the other subcontractors. They can't put a face to any of the names on the proposals . . . except yours. They remember you because you stood out. Your stutter made the conversation memorable, and since they remember you, they remember the discrepancy you caught that would have delayed the project and would've cost them a quarter of their markup. Your stutter was not a factor in their decision to accept your proposal, but your stutter put a face to the name on one of the several contracts in front of them.

That morning the woman you gave your number to decides to wear the coat she wore to the pub last Friday. Sliding her cell phone into her pocket, she feels a napkin and pulls it out and sees your number. She was approached by three men that night but she only remembers one. You were different. Not because you let her enjoy her night by not interrupting her "girls night" or because you didn't strike some obnoxious alpha posture to get her attention. She remembered you because you stuttered ordering your drink, owned it, and acknowledged her noticing it with self-acceptance. You were different and she liked that.

I'm not saying to use your stutter for attention. But the fact is that it attracts attention whether you like it or not. Trying to hide your stutter is a futile endeavor. Not only will it increase the severity of blocks but the stoic, soft spoken attitude that you are trying to convey will come across as inauthentic and paranoid. It's awkward for others who are trying to be polite as possible as they listen to you for them to pretend you don't stutter because *you're pretending* you don't stutter. Owning your stutter and allowing the stutter to pass naturally allows you to act naturally and your personality to come through as completely genuine.

That's your power: *the real you.*

Stuttering is a humanizing aspect of you. It makes you more relatable as a real person and eases the need others may feel to be "impressive" or false in any way. Because you come off as truly human, they can relax and do the same: *be human.*

Tough Love

15. Labels

It ain't what they call you.
It's what you answer to.
~W.C. Fields

We are labeled and we label ourselves as stutterers. This label can be attached to us in two ways. It can be something we are or something we possess. I am a stutterer or I have a stutter. Those perceptions exist simultaneously but embody different facets of our psyche. Both perceptions must be dealt with because each of them imposes its own burden, its own ponderous baggage.

To own your stutter, you must be able to carry it around with you effortlessly. Baggage is heavy, bulky and wastes your energy. You can't pretend to own your stutter, as much as you can't pretend to not be carrying any baggage. "Faking it" only comes off as awkward, feeds your insecurities, and eventually solidifies your false self-perceptions. Stuttering innately suppresses self-expression and programs the subconscious into believing that self-expression is not a good thing. It doesn't register the stutter as being the cause of negative responses; it falsely identifies any attempt at self-expression as the cause of negative feedback or detrimental self-perception.

I am a stutterer is a defining description of who you are. It's an involuntary state of being that you exist in. Because it is in relation to who you are, the shame incurred by the stutter during adolescence (imposed by the inaccurate perceptions of *others*) is attached to *who you are*, not how you speak. This is sometimes referred to as *toxic shame*.

Shame is not the same as embarrassment. Embarrassment is a response to something you have done, not to your persona or identity. *I have a stutter* is a self-describing label that elicits these feelings. *I have* means *to possess*. A stutter is *a thing*. It's yours. You own it. If you have an ugly car, you may feel embarrassed driving it, but it's yours, you own it. It's not an object of shame, but merely a source of embarrassment. Or not. You may love that car and not care what anyone thinks because you know your ugly car will start every morning without fail and cost you next to nothing to drive.

Shame is the belief that you are defective and undeserving. Shame is the biggest battle a stutterer will face. The self-belief that you are defective means that you are less valuable. That means all you have to do is become more valuable or make others less valuable to level the playing field right? Makes sense in theory but ... no, that's not how it works. Life isn't about rigging the value scales but getting rid of them all together. *To own your stutter* not only means you accept *having* (possessing) it, but you accept that having it is what makes you complete, real, *human*. You do this by forgiving yourself for disliking or hating yourself. Instead of a broken part of you, you have to see it as an aspect of your personality. When you *own your stutter* it's attractive to others because you are different but not projecting a need to be treated differently.

Shame projects itself onto others in the form of neediness, manipulation and pandering. To *own your stutter* is to stutter without shame. If your stutter is an attractive personality trait there is no reason to be ashamed of it. Understanding this and overcoming my own toxic shame was probably the most important thing I've ever done.

Shame cannot be removed because it actually doesn't exist. Shame is like darkness. Darkness doesn't exist. Darkness is the absence of light. To overcome darkness, you need to fill the space with light. By owning your stutter you illuminate the darkness of shame with the light of self-acceptance.

Earlier, I mentioned the need for accurate perspective. Changing your perspective about your stutter is the easiest way to achieve accurate perspective about the rest of your life, about *who you are.* I have amazing people in my life, authentic, beautiful, empathetic people who love me for who I am. I believe my stutter is the reason for this. I attract unique and quirky people because I am unique and possibly plenty quirky myself. I attract non-judgmental people because a judgmental person would not be able to comfortably share space with me.

Embarrassment is a complicated emotion with a simple solution. Relax... seriously just relax. Self-degradation is never a reasonable solution for anything, but laughing at yourself is. Embarrassment is simply the product of taking yourself too seriously. If you spill a glass of wine at the table the panic that ensues to contain the tsunami will trigger your body into fight or flight mode. Your face will get red. Your voice will tremble. You'll feel the eyes of the world staring directly at you with criticism, derision, even contempt.

But things like that happen in life, and at one time or another, they happen to everybody. Accidents *happen* and anybody with an ounce of life experience understands that. If you laugh at yourself, others laugh with you. Just like the rest of us, you're not perfect, and no one expects you to be.

Seriously, get over yourself and take off that diamond tiara with which you have foolishly crowned yourself. You're not the king or queen of anything, and nobody really cares that you're not.

I was talking to a client and I was bent over measuring something on their patio. He asked me a question and in my response I stuttered. As I stuttered, bent over, saliva drooled out of my mouth and onto my hand. Splat. I quickly wiped it off on my pantleg but I know he saw it. My face turned bright red, and an awkward silence ensued. The birds in the trees above us even shut up. I kept taking measurements and asked him something to break the silence, but I couldn't look at him in the eye. I rushed through the appointment and filled my hands with tools as I left so I could avoid the chance of an awkward and drool-damp handshake, and I made a hasty exit.

It's been over a month since that happened, and I still get a tight feeling in my chest when I think about it. It happened; there is nothing I can do to change it. I'm still embarrassed about it, even a month later. I could have saved myself a lot of discomfort If I would have just owned it. Instead of running away I could have said, "Wow, that's embarrassing." He probably would have agreed with me and moved on to discuss the details of the patio project. But I didn't own it in the moment and now I get to *own it forever*. It's like not paying a bill and being sent to collections. Instead of taking the initial small hit, you're stuck with accrued penalties and harassment and it's a long time to make it all go away.

If you *own your* stutter it's impossible for it to embarrasss you. The quickest way to genuinely *own your stutter* is to get over the fear of embarrassment. The only way to do that is to stutter with as many people in as many situations as possible. There's no other way around it. To own it is to be completely comfortable with it in any and all situations, without exception.

Go out in the world and talk. It may surprise you to see the severity of your stutter decline after immersing yourself in as many conversations as possible. The more you challenge the stutter, the more you reveal it, the less you fight it, the more comfortable you'll be...and the less you'll stutter. The stutter reacts to your efforts to fight it by fighting back. Let the damned thing do what it's going to do—stop fighting it—and let it ride off into the sunset.

16.
The Paradigm

It all begins and ends in your mind.
What you give power to has power over you.
~Pratibha Patil

The paradigm of a stutterer is that of constantly living a double life. On one hand you're an intelligent, capable, completely normal person. But on the other, you're intimidated by almost everything, tip-toeing through life to avoid conversations and everyday interactions. You're avoiding success and leadership opportunities out fear that you might have to stand up, take charge, and speak your mind.

While it's absolutely true that people don't care if you stutter, embracing that truth doesn't happen by simply flipping a switch. You need to experience that truth before you'll actually believe it, own it, and use it to set yourself free.

When I find myself feeling self-conscious, I remind myself it's coming from a place of unjustified fears. I remember what living in that paradigm cost me and then I regret not overcoming it sooner and that switch is quickly flipped.

Eight years ago I was the sole proprietor of a small construction company. I was invited to bid on a half-million-dollar contract to supply a new housing development with windows. Not to install them, not to warranty them, simply to supply them. Simple enough. Order them in phases over six months and schedule delivery. I wrote the proposal in which I would very likely net a $30,000 profit, simply for doing little more than routine paperwork. The general contractor was looking for small veteran-owned businesses to work with so they'd get government rebates and tax incentives on their ledgers. Since I was the only qualified and licensed sub-contractor with the qualifications, I was a shoo-in.

You're going to think I'm crazy, but this was my mental state at the time: I actually paid people to talk on the phone for me. I'd type everything out and let them talk. The phone didn't ring too often for me to handle incoming calls, but I'd let the answering machine pick them up whenever I was in the office alone. If I won this contract, I would have to attend weekly meetings and give verbal presentations in front of city hall planners, all the other subcontractors, and possibly the local media.

So what did I do? I declined the invitation. My finished proposal sat in my hard drive like a treasure chest at the bottom of the ocean. How crazy is that? I understand why I did it. I know the truth, but I don't like it. What if I'd been awarded that contract and had to give those presentations? I would have occasionally stood in front of a room full of people and stuttered into a microphone. Realistically, what's the worst that would have happened? It would've been a room full of professionals. In all likelihood, nothing would have happened at all. No one would have cared that it took me a little longer to get my words out, and the additional income I would've received could have catapulted my business to the next level. What exactly was I so scared of? It made zero sense to reject that invitation because of stage fright. So what did actually happen?

    I had three employees, two apprentices and a part-time secretary. I worked about ten hours a day and eight of them were doing physical labor. That was my comfort zone. I didn't have to talk much, I could work with my hands, and my craftsmanship spoke for me. As a small-time contractor that is all I had to do. Stay in my comfort zone. I always did the job right the first time so I didn't have to explain anything while employees handled the phones. If I expanded the company, my daily duties would have revolved around the office and running the business. That would've meant more phone calls from people that needed to speak to the owner. It would've consisted of speaking in front of people several times a week and attending meetings where covert stuttering and word replacement would not be suitable. Trade talk is specific, synonyms for technical words are not readily available and using them would be confusing.

I lived in the paradigm of a stutterer. My career, relationships and self-esteem were dependent upon my ability to avoid situations in which I was expected to speak on command. If I could get a rhythm in my head while tapping my foot, and launch the sound off the back of my throat at the point of near full exhalation, I could force out a sentence with minimal blocking. That is nearly impossible to do on command or while dodging impromptu questions. Answering a predictable question ahead of time required a suffocating sequence of vowel-less phrases, an awkward and exhausting survival mechanism.\

All of this might seem logical because eventually I had to communicate and devise techniques to speak or I was going to go broke. So I constantly found verbal loopholes, always struggling to become part of the "normal" communication going on around me.

It was exhausting. I needed another option. It wasn't a new trail I had to blaze or an unforgiving hostile new frontier I had to conquer. It was a well-traveled path, and anyone who is successful and acknowledges their own "imperfection" has walked it. I could have simply *owned it*. Instead of taking ten seconds to breathe, tap my foot, and word switch my way through a sentence, I could've taken ten seconds longer and said what I needed to stay, with stutter and all.

It's taken me losing everything to understand the reality, *my reality*: I stutter, I don't block, stumble, repeat, choke, drool or seize. I just *stutter*. When I block, stumble, repeat, choke, drool and seize, it's because *I pretend I don't stutter*. If I *owned* my stutter, if I was comfortable with my stutter and didn't try not to stutter; I would barely stutter. I wasn't afraid of stuttering in front of my fiancée, kid, waiter, customer or the news cameras at City Hall. I was afraid of *blocking, stumbling, and seizing* on camera at city hall. How twisted is that? My inability to own my stutter and allow it to simply be part of my overall persona forced me to adopt self-defeating defense mechanisms that torpedoed any success I could have had.

Consider that for a moment. I would've preferred to have a mini-seizure rather than stutter. I would've rather failed in life masquerading as normal, than to have succeeded as a businessman with a speech impediment?

How insane is that?

Well...actually it's not insane at all. It's the point of this book. It's the reason I've studied and researched and obsessively dissected the complete paradigm of stuttering.

The stuttering, awkward, handicapped, autistic or developmentally disabled kid who is the outcast in his adolescence and would give anything to just be normal will grow up with the same shame, stigma and self-hate that led me to the Big Sur bridge one rainy night with the hope that I might escape my own existence.

Exile is a legitimate fear as a child. It is programmed into our DNA to be accepted into society and to survive daily hazards encountered by our ancestors. To be exiled from the group was to be vulnerable to predators, enemies and starvation. Those fears are real to our subconscious minds. Our fear of being different is actually our fear of death..

Why are we afraid of heights? We can look down at the top of a skyscraper over a secure railing without the danger of falling and our body's hormonal responses go wild, with adrenaline leading the charge into full-blown terror. It's just natural, as our subconscious brain tells us to be careful. When success is at your doorstep and you have to choose to leave the safety of the village and forge your own trail, your inner caveman becomes stressed, uncomfortable. When your brain and self-image evolve in constant fear of exile, you'll do anything in your power to disguise whatever it is that makes you different. Many people figure this out early in life and thrive as individuals. Others, like myself; have to hit rock bottom before they realize the only thing trying to feed them to the wolves is their ego.

17.
Kids & Parents

Accept the challenges so that you can feel the exhilaration of victory.
~General George S. Patton

For any child—especially a young stutterer—approval, validation, and encouragement are vital to emotional development and well-being. Once a belief has taken root in young minds it is a difficult task to reframe future situations which positively resemble previous ones. We are creatures of habit, habits become lifestyles, and our lifestyles produce our outcomes.

My school didn't provide speech therapy, so my Mom fought for it. She refused to let them put me in remedial classes just because I couldn't speak fluently, and she tried her best to protect me from the harassment of other kids. She did the best she could with the pre-internet era's limited information and resources. She reminded me to slow down and breathe, and she never rushed me or belittled me. My parents were "tough love" parents, but they loved me unconditionally. They sacrificed their wants for my needs and always treated me as if I didn't stutter. I was punished for misbehaving and praised for my achievements. They made sure I knew that my stutter had nothing to do with my intelligence or my ability to succeed in anything.

We always had enough money to live comfortably, but eating out and new shoes were luxuries. I loved pizza, and my parents couldn't really afford to have it delivered on a regular basis. But I could have pizza whenever I wanted. All I had to do was pick up the phone and...order it. That was tough love in practice. In today's world, my parents would have been accused of child abuse, but it taught me a lesson: if I wanted something, I'd have to work for it. My folks just acted like they had no doubts I could do it so my real reward was the achievement itself. For that, I'm beyond thankful.

In elementary school, my stutter was severe. I couldn't complete a full sentence if my life depended on it. My entire body would lock up when I blocked, hands would curl in and my mouth would get stuck wide open. I had to use my hand to close it sometimes. I had no control over my body once I started to speak. I tried to make that call for pizza many times. I would practice for hours but "Hello" took me at least a minute to say. So placing the pizza order, complete with return phone number and our address were like climbing Mt. Everest barefoot.

The kitchen window faced west. I'd watch the sunset through it while standing by the phone. The phone was on the wall back then, and I was all of four feet tall. My mom would lean against the kitchen counter, watching as I often chickened out and lost the inner battle. Sometimes the people at the pizza place would say "Hello?" five times and hang up before I could even make a sound. That was scary to me because I thought they were mad at me. I looked up at Mom and she inhaled deeply, exhaled calmly with "Hello." Just like my speech therapist taught me. I followed her lead, breathed in, exhaled, prolonging the H and failed a few times before I got it right. When I finally did, I perked up, and she smiled. I was standing at the base of Mt. Everest as I reached up for the phone, put it to my ear, and dialed. I had the number memorized by then, but dialed slowly. I was breathing: in through my nose and out through my mouth. The ring tone snapped me back to reality. I froze. All of my blood rushed to my head, my throat clenched itself tight and I was paralyzed in fear. I looked up at my mother, terrified. She inhaled deeply and exhaled saying,"Hello."

  They answered. I panicked but didn't run away. I made some kind of inaudible utterance that sounded like "hello," breathed in as much air as I could ,and before they could hang up, I yelled in a high pitched prepubescent voice, "I stutter!" The young lady on the other line replied with a smile in her voice. "Okay, how may I help you?" I still remember her voice, she giggled but not mockingly, it was more of a 'how cute' giggle. I could hear the noisy pizza parlor in the background ,but she was silent for what was probably ten minutes while I blocked and stumbled my way through the order, return phone number, and address. (That lady is still a hero to me and I never knew what she even looked like.)

I hung the phone up and felt a wave of indestructability and self-esteem course through my body like a super hero. I'd reached the summit of the highest mountain in the world ,and standing on top of it was my mom. Her eyes were watering and her smile had an angelic softness to it. I remember that smile because I saw that smile again when I was 22, boarding a bus with 60 other recruits heading off to war. I don't remember what she said at that time, but I remember how her voice trembled. Her pride for me when I ordered that pizza was so deep I could feel the energy. I felt the same energy from her when I boarded that bus too.

That phone call to me was life changing; everything became possible . For my mother, that phone call had been a moment of amazing grace. She had put the work in, she'd fought for me, and she deserved that victory. Needless to say, as my family sat around the table smiling at me eating that pizza out of a cardboard box, that was the best meal I ever had.

My Dad never mentioned my stutter. It's not that he was ashamed of me or in denial about my stutter. He's a *life's not fair, suck it up* kind of guy so I think he was worried I'd have a harder life because of my speech. Making him proud has always been a factor in my decisions. He's my stepdad, but he worked hard to support me and raised me as his own. He is a man of habit, does what he does and does it consistently. I don't remember him ever calling in sick at work or complaining about any ailment. He'd go to his construction job with joints swollen twice their size and limp back into the house after dark, covered in sawdust and metal shavings. I have nothing but admiration for him and love him with all my heart. I know he feels the same way about me, but at times when I was growing up it was hard to tell. He always introduced me as his son with pride but looked down nervously as I spoke. If we were having a conversation and I took too long he would sigh like he was frustrated. It used to hurt me because I took it as disappointment. Today, as I learn to reframe my past and see things in a less judgmental way, I understand a few things. He wasn't embarrassed or disappointed; he was helpless. He would have given anything to help me with my stutter and he did. Speech therapy cost my parents a fortune. I did more than my share of acting out in anger, so missing work once a week to pick me up from the principal's office or the police station was a serious burden.

What I perceived as his disappointment in me was his frustration that he couldn't save me. Parents do that. They internalize any problem their children have and blame themselves for their inability to help. Even if it's a condition medical science can't figure out, they expect themselves to find the answers.

My Dad made sure I knew how to work hard, support myself ,and function as a contributing member of society. He taught me what he knew the only way he knew how. My relationship with my parents today is stronger than it has ever been. When I decided to live as if I don't stutter, refused to blame my stutter for my addictions and relationship problems, wean myself off of the sympathy trip and fail forward without the comfort of a handicap net, they saw the change in me and knew that I was going to be alright. I freed myself from the prison in my mind and consequently freed them from the burden of their guilt.

If we stuttering adults do not fully spread our wings and seek complete independence and self-sufficiency, we keep our parents in captivity as our safety net. No one is homeless, helpless or hopeless because they stutter. There are always other issues at work. I promise that if you are honest and address the real issues in your life, your speech will improve simply because stuttering does not exist where it is not needed.

Let me say that again; *Stuttering does not exist where it is not needed.*

If I could give the parent of a stutterer any advice, it would be to follow my parents' example of "tough love." I know it sounds harsh because the stuttering voice of their child naturally spurs compassion in the parental heart, but "tough love" is two words.

Love is the objective. Love is an enabler but "tough love" is a motivator. The child feels like an outcast. He or she is alone in this battle and you can't change that. It is a solo mission and they have to take point and deal with the enemy one-on-one. Always walk behind them on that journey, encourage, compliment and let them know you have nothing but faith in their abilities to do anything. Obviously speech therapy is a great source for tools but the real cure is *confidence*. You know that they are capable of doing anything that any other kid their age can do. Give them the encouragement to explore their skills, talents and passions. My friend's son began stuttering and his folks got him into speech therapy right off the bat, which helped considerably. The boy's father asked me what he should do at home. I told him "Nothing. He's a normal boy, treat him like he is." His son can hit three-pointers from across the street. They play ball and have fun. He's doing just fine.

My children do not stutter but I feel guilt and self-blame for any situation they are in that they can't handle. I feel as if I've failed because it was my job to teach them how to deal with everything that's out there in this unpredictable world. My daughter is older and on her own now, and I feel as if I messed up as a parent on a million different levels. Of course, she laughs at my concern and blows off my validation requests. She knows I'm fishing for a compliment and gives me "cookies" sparingly. I've asked her a few questions about what it's been like growing up with a dad that stuttered. Her answers have been as beautiful and intelligent as she is. Her grandparents on her mom's side were from the Philippines. When she was young, she thought my stutter was an accent like her grandparents'. She had no idea I stuttered until someone told her.

I used to order a cheeseburger with no cheese whenever I took my daughter out. She thought I was just being funny, and didn't realize I couldn't say words that start with the letter H, "hamburger" being the one in question.

She said that my stutter was humanizing. She's grateful she got to see her dad in that light because kids often idolize their parents and feel insufficient. But my daughter understands that her tough GI-Joe dad has flaws, and that has allowed her to be more comfortable in her own skin.

My son—now a teenager—experienced a traumatic incident as a child and he does his best to cope with it. He is a loving kid. He gives affection freely and loves people. At 13 he was preparing three-course meals which could easily have been five-courses if I'd allowed it. Watching a natural talent manifest itself through your child is an amazing experience. Cooking is therapy for him and I can't wait to watch him graduate culinary school someday. He had a tough time in elementary and middle school. He's somewhat socially awkward and has had a hard time making friends. He was six when the stars aligned and I met his mom and I got the chance to become his dad.

I wince at the mistakes I made through the years as a father. I tried so hard to act like my own father that I was never actually in the moment with my son. I spent more time trying to indoctrinate than communicate. But we've shared things that no one else can understand. We have a perfect connection of "imperfectness".

He went to the same school I did, and he had a hard time just like I did. I growled every time I stepped on that campus remembering what happened in my own childhood on that playground. My son didn't have many friends in school. His demeanor got him bullied and he acted out in frustration. (Sound familiar?) He escaped the world in his own little LegoLand. He was so obsessed with Legos that I had to check his pockets every morning because he would play with them during class. His mom had to pick him up from school one day because he was hysterical. He had smuggled a few Lego people in his backpack and the teacher took them away from him. He broke down and became so distraught that he couldn't control himself. That afternoon, sitting with him in the school principal's office, we asked him why he took them to school when he knew he wasn't supposed to. Almost a decade later his response still devastates me: "They're my only friends…"

My heart has never been more broken than when he said those words. As a stutterer who went to the same school, who experienced childhood trauma, who saw what he was going through, I'd failed him.

I was still at a point in my own life where I was the victim. If I had a unique personality trait that I wore like a badass scar instead of a sympathy-starved affliction, I could have been a rock for him. I didn't speak up for him in the principal's office that day because I was embarrassed to stutter. I didn't call the school when he told me he was being bullied because his mom made all the phone calls. I was a coward hiding behind a stutter, and I failed my son at that point because I was a full grown elephant who still hadn't figured out how to get a stick out the ground.

Owning your stutter, reframing your past ,and refusing sympathy are not pseudo-science bumper sticker slogans. Your child's development cannot exceed your own if they are still in your care. They grow in your space and your space can only be as nurturing and stable as you are. I did not let him down because I stutter. I let him down because I was co-dependent, insecure and self-loathing. My stutter was an excuse to be that way, and nobody could tell me otherwise.

My son is growing up fast. He's taller than his mom now and will probably be looking down at me soon. I have a lot of work to do to get where I need to be for both of us. He grew up watching his mom order my food and make my phone calls. He watched me get frustrated when I couldn't communicate what I wanted to and instead hosted my own pity parties. I owe it to him to be a secure successful stutterer so he can navigate this life and blaze his own trail with courage and integrity. If he's still awkward when he grows up, he'll be awkward on his own terms and carry his badass scar with pride and self acceptance.

All parents struggle with inadequacy. None of us knows what we're doing. We're just doing the best we can with what we have. We are all teaching our kids what we know, the only way we know how. I did my best and I know you're doing the same. No amount of reading, research or advice can prepare you to succeed in raising your unique, one-in-a-seven-billion child.

We wake up every day to new challenges. We go to sleep every night with regrets and the occasional win. Every kid is different, and there is no standard operating manual to refer to. My sister has two masters degrees in Human Development, both of her kids have a filing cabinet full of academic awards, and even she plays it by ear on a day-to-day basis. The only way you can fail as a parent is to not try and the only way to fail at trying is to have an excuse why you didn't.

Tough Love

18.
Self-expression

*Belief has the power to change your
inner state and your outer world.*
                              ~J.P. Warren

Modern-day psychologists believe that 90% of what we communicate is nonverbal. The words we actually say account for about 7% of what we communicate to others. Remember when I said body language will change your game?

Consider these two scenarios...

1. You're at a job interview, and your stutter setting is turned up because you're nervous. But you already had a phone interview and they called you back. They knew you stuttered in the phone interview and they called you back, so it's time to let them get to know you. You're sitting in the chair, leaning forward with your hands together, fingers interlaced, legs crossed at the ankles, slouching. They ask you about your experience, strengths and weaknesses. You want them to like you. You answer as politely and quickly as

possible in a soft tone, hoping to camouflage the severity of your stutter. They ask you directly if you feel comfortable talking on the phone. You say yes, tapping your feet against each other and make a second of eye contact before you look back down, pretending to read the job summary they've handed you. They thank you for your time, stand up and shake your hand. You thank them, bowing your head as you make a B-line to the door. They send you an email a few days later stating the position has been filled. *Dammit, your stutter cost you another job.* If only you'd breathed out your words better or had rolled your consonants more smoothly you totally would've been hired. Your more than qualified for the gig, but you stutter...

Or...

2. You're at a job interview, and your stutter setting is turned up that day because you're nervous, but you already had a phone interview and they called you back. You're sitting in the chair, shoulders back with your elbows on the armrests, legs relaxed, shoulder-width apart. They ask you about your experience, strengths and weaknesses. You want them to like you and you answer as professionally as possible, in an enthusiastic tone. They knew you stuttered in the

phone interview and they called you back, so it's time to let them get to know you. They ask you directly if you feel comfortable talking on the phone. You say you do, with a smile while making eye contact with them. "My stutter is turned up today, I get nervous at job interviews." They smile and respond in kind, "Doesn't everybody…" You genuinely laugh because you know it's true. They thank you for your time, stand up and shake your hand. You thank them for the opportunity, calling them by their names and smile as you calmly exit the office. They send you an email a few days later offering you the position.

Quite a different outcome, isn't it?

In the second scenario, you obviously fooled them and tricked your way into getting hired. Or did you? You won't fool anyone if you try to fake it. Only if you're truly comfortable with your stutter and come across as genuine will you come across as authentic and trustworthy, a key qualification for every employment situation. You need to achieve a genuine comfort level with your stutter so that you come across as *a real person,* not as someone trying to hide something.

Prospective employers aren't judging your fluency levels. They're judging your sincerity and trustworthiness. They don't want to have to walk on eggshells around you or worry about catering to your handicap. If you're not walking on eggshells about it or sensitive about it, then it quickly becomes irrelevant to their hiring decision. If you don't consider it a handicap, then it isn't a handicap.

Body language is how people judge you as soon as you walk into the room. People do not feel comfortable around people who physically close themselves off to the world or act submissively. You can learn to fake it from any pick-up artist but that will only erode your self esteem even further. When you fake it—when you pretend to be something you're not—you're actually revealing your false persona and implying a certain level of dishonesty lurking in your character. Truth and trust go hand-in-hand. They come from the inside. Without that truth, any attempts to portray confidence or sincerity come off as merely false.

It all starts with an inner *belief* in who you are. And you can only *believe* who you are when you are *real* and admit who you are *to yourself.* That inner belief gives you the power to act subconsciously, honestly, and transparently. When you're *real,* you have nothing to hide.

It must be a subconscious reaction to situations. How do you make yourself do something without making yourself do something? You do the same thing you did during speech therapy. You practice speaking as you exhale until your body does it by itself, without consciously forcing it. When you brush your teeth or drive your car, you're not concentrating on every movement. You've done it so many times that it's just a part of your muscle memory. When your body is closed off to the world, when you're not being true to the *true you* that you know, you're sending off signals: *caution*.

It might seem like being timid or shy is a good thing, and that people will think you're nice and friendly, but it's actually interpreted by others as fearful. If someone is fearful of social interaction, they have shame, guilt, or lies they haven't dealt with. Friends will be a little more forgiving of this, but romantic partners and employers don't want to gamble on whether or not there is a personality behind your carefully constructed false front. Shame isn't self-imposed and being timid isn't a bad thing. It may be your state at the moment, where you're at mentally in life, and its neither good nor bad. It just needs to be dealt with, resolved, and overcome.

Overcoming shame and opening yourself up to the world is difficult because you're allowing yourself to be vulnerable. If you're frightened, you clam up so you can take a hit and protect your vitals. It takes a lot of courage to take a hit with your arms spread out and chin up. But that's exactly what you have to do. Approaching situations with your arms spread and chin out (with an open heart) is certainly not easy, but the rewards are invaluable. If you stutter without hiding it, sitting in a crowded space taking up as much room as you need to be comfortable, and admit the things you're ashamed of, something magical happens.

Nothing happens. Nothing at all. That's what is truly amazing. You quickly learn that what you were afraid of is possible, but not probable. If you stutter, you're not going to get beaten up or mocked on the schoolyard. If you sit up straight and spread your shoulders, no one is gonna challenge you like some uncaged alpha gorilla. You're going to feel confident over time, and before long *you will be confident.* Admitting shame is sometimes all it takes to switch your mindset from *I'm in hell* to *Hell* to *Hell yeah!* It's as simple as saying it to someone: "I'm ashamed of my stutter and wish I could just own it."

I promise you this: Whomever you say that to has something about themselves that erodes their confidence as well. They feel the same way you do about *something* and once you open your heart to them, they'll do the same. Before you know it, both of you will have discovered a new sense of freedom and you'll begin to truly *communicate.* This is how trust erupts to build confidence and friendships.

If you need to, tell everyone you meet that you stutter. Seriously, I did it for a week and I think my blood pressure actually changed. I started every conversation with, "I stutter, give me a sec" or something similar. Be open, be vulnerable, say aloud what you're worried about, and enjoy the freedom. Your entire demeanor will change. Once you open yourself up inside, your body follows suit. People will actually ask you about your stutter with genuine interest instead of side-stepping what may be an obvious reality for you.

I actually like it when people ask me about my stutter. My answers might make them uncomfortable but they never bother me because they are *true*. It's often my calling card to connect with people on a personal *human* level. It's my source of creativity and empathy. I smile when people ask about my stutter and I tell them, "It's just my thing, I was born with it."

Open body language and vulnerability reveal our true personality. We as stutterers have issues expressing ourselves vocally. Our personalities, attitudes, opinions, and our unique intelligence can be veiled in the eyes of those around us by our speech blocks. I personally love telling jokes, but can't nail a punch line to save my life. It's like a trigger for me. I'm right there: Three guys walk into a bar. Time for the punchline. BLOCK, ugh.

We also have issues with asserting ourselves or expressing a point of view. That's because deep inside, we feel like we're not taken seriously when we speak directly or confrontationally. If you're expressing anger or disappointment, the energy of your sentiment dissipates if you have to start over or pause to breathe. It can be disheartening and make you feel like you can't really stand up for yourself. This may seem like a hopeless situation, and in some ways, it is. It really is. There is no way around it. To express yourself clearly and forcefully, one needs to be reasonably fluent physically and verbally. To be more fluent in those respects, you have to be willing and able to express yourself. Hollywood movies have traditionally portrayed stutterers as timid and stupid because audiences have been conditioned to interpret characters using that manner of speech as indicative of low IQ or cowardice It's our stereotype and the only way to change it is to disprove it. When the drill sergeant asked if I was scared of him because I stuttered, he was projecting that same clichéd stereotype. When I told him I wasn't afraid of him but that I stuttered, I was separating the stutter from the stereotype.

If you stutter when you speak but conduct yourself with self respect, your actions will always speak louder than your words.

19.
The Quick Fix Fallacy

Instant gratification takes too long.
~Carrie Fisher

*H*ello I'm Shane, and I'm a member of the instant-gratification fad diet generation.
Remember when fats were the devil, carbs were Hitler, your mom did Tae Bo in the living room and gluten made it to the seventh level of Dante's inferno?

Pepperidge Farms remembers because you dipped them in ice cream watching *The Biggest Loser* on TV and loathed Mondays because that's when you were always starting your diet. Monday always came and you woke up to the smell of coffee brewing in the kitchen next to the capsule dispenser filled with a week's worth of ginsing, green tea, and ginko.

And now the cold shower and skin tightening cream jolts you awake and launches your metabolism into Beast Mode. You've created your own reality show, in which you'll walk across the stage in your god bod. Freed from the tyranny of fat you see yourself practicing your right to bare arms . . . and shoulders, sliding into the spaghetti-strap tanktop that came with the 20-lb barrel of pure hydrolyzed whey protein isolate. Creatine monohydrate now courses through your veins, the magic bullet screaming the war cry of your tribe, *NoFear!* and diluting the only carbs you'll be allowed to ingest for the rest of the day. Driving to work your hands shake, gripping tight to your reusable earth-friendly glass water bottle with the fold- out straw that's hard to clean. Your hands grip tighter, calming their quake as the beast inside you explodes with jitters because your fat- burner pills had 325mgs of caffeine and you knocked them down your throat with coconut milk and coffee.

You pull into the employee parking lot, turning off the *Stop Stuttering in 30 Days* CD you got from that guy on Youtube who put vowels over binary beats at 423.67 hertz.

The break room in the office with the donuts is a hazard zone to be consciously avoided. You've prepared a Spartan warrior's diet for the day and walk around the block during lunch while consuming sodium free, grain fed, skinless chicken breast in a lettuce tortilla. Your body is twitching from metabolism boosters and your heart is turbocharged, red-lining the tach at your track speed of 3 miles per hour.

Then, back to work, the tremors subside and your body chemistry balances itself out as you zero-carb crash in a corner. It's the bosses birthday, so you pretend you care as you eyeball the grocery store cake and generic Neapolitan ice cream (everybody likes different flavors even if it all blends together because the scooper is too big). But you're a Spartan. The motivational video said so and so you self-righteously deny yourself the joys of all those weak (but normal) people around you.

These folks have no idea that as you sing *Happy Birthday* your voice is reverberating in your ear because the Stop Stuttering Hearing Aid is so incognito. These people who are so blind to your cleverness don't realize they'll all soon be reporting directly to you, just as soon as you master your tongue and chisel your bod. You're going to have six-pack abs and be able to say those words without endlessly stammering out the S, the P, the O, or the A.

Then, the day's work is done. *It's go time!* you announce, punching the time clock. Fist clenched, you walk up to your car in the parking lot like you want to fight and *beep-beep* it into submission. Removing your work shirt, you cover the tanktop with a t-shirt because you know you can't rock spaghetti straps without cleanly-defined deltoids. Twenty minutes later, you step into the gym. The smell of rubber mats, mildewed showers, and sweaty clothes overtake your senses as you prepare for battle.

Then it happens, kryptonite. You forgot your headphones at home and don't have time to drive across town and back because in just an hour your online chatroom is discussing the struggle of speaking to automated phone systems. You could always press *zero* to talk to a live representative, but they might shame you by saying hello twice before you can utter a sound, so that's not an option.

Okay, you'll just have to start the gym thing tomorrow.

Two weeks in, you feel like you're dying and have the temperament of a feral cat . . . but you lost four whole pounds of water. The three total hours at the gym are paying off!

And then it's break time. Your cheat day is here. You've earned it, and feast you will. You spend the weekend consuming 12,000 calories of anything you can get your hands on, because your body is in survival mode and doesn't give a shit about your god-bod visualization exercises. Your body chemistry is so jacked you don't have the energy to do anything and before long you just give up. The anti-stutter mix tape puts you to sleep and the earpiece hurts. You feel like you're speaking better, but between the carbo-starved diet and the half-assed gym sessions, you've been so irritable when speaking to anyone whether or not any of this "system" has worked is up for a vote.

Facts are facts. Your speech impediment is not a spiritual, metaphysical, or hypothetical part of you. It's a physical manifestation of the chemical reactions and synapses firing in your highly complex physical brain. Increasing your fluency is no different than increasing your metabolism or learning another language. There is simply no quick fix. If there were effective systems, therapies, or medical protocols, some pharmaceutical conglomerate would own it and be printing money marketing it to the millions of us who stutter. Your body learns a skill by rote.

Repetition.

Practice.

Muscle memory.

Training.

All of which require you to *get out of your comfort zone* and work hard enough so that the discomfort becomes tolerable. Continue working past the plateau of "tolerable," and the pain is replaced by a feeling of accomplishment, fulfillment, mastery.

There is no quick way to become a master at anything. Ask Tiger Woods or Pete Sampras or Eric Clapton or . . . you get the idea. Champions never stop practicing, never stop struggling for mastery, never stop pushing out of their comfort zones, never stop working.

Quick fixes are a myth, a fallacy promulgated by the world of marketing. Your brain was trained to stutter or to fight your stutter over a long period of time. You may have mastered it by now, to the point where it's "easy" to stutter and nearly impossible not to.

The challenge is to get out of that comfort zone and do the hard work it takes to retrain and reboot your system. Sure, you can drop a few pounds in one week or speak more clearly in two weeks by shocking your system into temporary compliance, but you don't need "temporary." Your body will bounce right back into old patterns, you'll put the pounds right back on where they were, and your speech will degrade into its habitual patterns the minute you dare to let up, look the other way, or try to avoid the practice, the pain, and the *work*.

Long term fluency requires mental fitness. Mental fitness requires a regimen of stress and rest just like the voluntary muscles of your body do.

Go talk in public. Meet and greet new people. Attack your blocking words head-on. Make phone calls, feel the burn. Give yourself a headache, the shakes, and cold sweats. Embrace the anxiety. Push yourself. Challenge your mental faculties. Face the fear. Let the embarrassment wash over you. Then stop. Rest. Not too long. Be your own coach, exhorting yourself from the sidelines to *get out there and kick some ass*.

Now do it again. Rinse and repeat. Over and over and over. Tough love? You bet. But it is *love*.

And love conquers all.

20. Normal

If you are always trying to be normal,
You will never know how amazing you can be.
~Maya Angelou

About a year ago I was working on a project and lost all inspiration. In an attempt to summon the muses, I figured I'd do what writers are supposed to do.

I went to a coffee shop. I sat in the corner with my back to the wall, laid my notebook on the table and sipped my coffee with my temple resting on my index finger. Because . . . uh, that's what writers do, right?

It wasn't busy but there were at least 20 people in the café. People came and went, some laughed, some rushed, some were writers too because they were there with their index finger pressed against their heads like *shoot me*. The door opened and a woman entered. She didn't look around like everyone usually did upon entering. Arms crossed, and on a mission to the register, she marched to the line and stood there, regiment-ready. My first impression of her was pretty negative. Her demeanor was cold and shut off to the world. *Bitchy* would be the best description.

Outside of the café in the parking lot, there were three guys leaning against a car, watching her through the storefront. As I scanned the café, everyone was looking at her. The people working there were even eyeing her. Everybody in the joint was focused on her, and I don't mean like casually, but staring. She must have noticed, but her eyes didn't thoughtlessly scan the room while waiting in line like most people do. Stutterers know the feeling when people are looking you and they think you don't notice. She just stared at the menu. I let it go and returned to my one-finger writer's salute.

The guys in the parking lot were sitting on an old Chevelle, and I had a brain flash about writing a piece about classic cars and why men love them; brute force and metallic finesse. I never wrote it, but it still sounded cool. I've actually never written anything of value in a coffee shop. I'm not even sure it's possible for a writer to get anything worthwhile done sitting in a coffee shop.

I was looking at the car and noticed the guys stiffen up, their heads all pointed the same way, so mine did too. The bitchy chick in line was now walking toward the back of the café where I was, and It hit me. I realized why everyone in the place was looking at her: she was stunning.

Then the reality hit me. Every eye in the room was on her as she sat down at a table with two chairs, placing her purse on one of them and then rummaging through it. Then she looked in my direction and we caught each other's eye. Her eyes were kind; I could see a gentle soul behind them. She asked me if she could use my pen. It was in my mouth so I chuckled no, but reached in my backpack for another one. She walked over and thanked me with a laugh. As she returned to her seat, I began to feel annoyed by everyone staring at her. I reprimanded myself internally for my superficial judgement of her and locked eyes with a guy across the café who quickly looked down and then back to her. When your own daughter is that age it bothers you...

What would it feel like to have people staring at you all the time? The guys on the car had a hawk's gaze on her and people inside the café stopped talking when she walked past. It would probably be a constant feeling of discomfort and self-consciousness. If the attention given an attractive woman is this obvious in a coffee shop, what is it like in a crowded place with hundreds of people? How does someone with such kind eyes have such a cold demeanor? I realized that as an average-looking stuttering man approaching middle age, I had the same insecurity standing in line at a coffee shop as a 20-something year-old beautiful young woman.

In restaurants, I order whatever I want no matter how long it takes, but I still feel the attention of others if I get hung up on a word. It's short-lived, a few seconds or so, and then everything goes back to "normal." I've stuttered, placed my order, and then...it's over.

But for this gorgeous young woman, dealing with attention from strangers is a constant, a fact of life for her. Like a damp, heavy fog, the discomfort we stutterers feel in those fleeting moments only lifts for her when she's alone. You might argue that it's good attention, but I don't think being gawked at or provoking silence with your mere presence feels very good.

We want to speak more fluently because we appreciate and even revere smooth speech. We want to be more attractive because we idolize attractive people. People are more than voices and faces. Our outside physical appearance and our voices are such a minute aspect of who we really are. Any part of us that is even marginally outside the norm of society is judged as our whole. It doesn't matter if it's a stutter like mine or a guarded posture like this young woman's. Her demeanor did not match the personality in her smile. When all eyes are on us, I guess it's normal to try to deflect that unwanted attention.

When all ears are on us, we do the same thing. We close ourselves off to the world and our demeanor becomes guarded. We forsake who we are and become someone we're not to deflect attention from anything that deviates from what we consider to be normal. What's *normal*? What level of attractiveness is normal? What age, income, race, or religion is normal? Mathematically, you can calculate demographics, but they vary on the next city block. If the woman in the coffee shop made a median income for her age in her city is she *normal*? Apparently not, because she caught everyone's attention. Therefore, regardless of every other statistic, she's not normal. What if she wasn't attractive? Is *that* normal? Is unattractive normal? If people don't stutter are they normal as long as they don't reach a certain level of physical symmetry?

Nobody is "normal," and even if they could be normal in the eyes of one person, there are a couple billion people on the planet who consider something else normal.

If there is no "normal" and everybody has some personal trait that generates undesired attention, then that part of them is *normal* because it is the only thing we all have.

Therefore, *your stutter is the only thing normal about you.*

It's a beautiful concept. The only thing we all have in common is the thing we hide from each other the most. Stop hiding it. Be who you are as a whole and stop covering it up with someone you're not.

Tough Love

21.
It Can Be Funny

Find out who you are and be that person.
~Ellen DeGeneres

True story:
There's a guy at work named Robert who prefers to be called Bob. Bob writes his name as Robert, so people naturally call him that. But when people call him Robert he says, "B-O-B, Bob." Guys make everything a joke in their circle so we started calling him B-O-B-Bob, which became BBB-Bob. My boss walked in the shop looking for Bob and yelled BBB-Bob. I turned the corner and said "What the fuck boss, I'm calling the ADA!" My boss is an awesome guy, but has the kind of job that makes your head spin so sometimes it takes a second for him to get the jokes. He looked at me like the Department of Political Correctness was going to dispatch SEAL Team Six and shut down our whole operation. "Shane, shit, I didn't mean…" I'm laughing, BBB-Bob is laughing and my boss, being a stand up guy who would never make fun of anyone for anything, feels like shit. I apologetically told him I was kidding as he walked back in

his office and I headed to my inbox to check my manifest for the day.

I think every day should start out with a good joke.

Just for the record, I'm guilty of being a pain in the ass to work for or to manage. I stutter but for some reason, I speak Fluent sarcasm. Here's an example of what I'm talking about:

I'm looking over work orders on the morning I'm scheduled to meet with a client who is deaf. My sense of humor begins doing cartwheels through a poppy field. The work orders state in bold, italic, underlined, all caps letters: **<u>SHE IS DEAF AND READS LIPS</u>** . I turn to Bob, slide the work order toward him and point to the note. Bob and I are good friends; he knows he has a pass on any good stutter jokes but never has any. I look at him, he looks at me, clueless. I say, "She damn sure won't see this one coming." Bob freezes for a second, and as it sinks in he buries his face in his hands, bright red with laughter.

I arrive at the client's house, still giddy from the morning's hysterics. I'm a professional and understand that some jokes may be funny in the shop but are inappropriate in front of clients. I am also not familiar with deaf people, so I don't know what is offensive to them or not. I mean what is the equivalent of *Did you forget your name?* to deaf people? I don't freaking know.

The house is on a narrow one-way street, so I pull my truck onto the sidewalk in the only place it will fit. I'd only be there for a short time, so I figure Phoenix cops have better things to do. I proceed to her front door, straight-faced and all business. I knock. Her dog is watching me through the window and I can see her sitting on the back porch. Her dog watches me approach, waits for me to knock, then runs to her, sits and looks at the front door, waiting. Watching. Guarding.

I'm watching this in awe. Her dog told her that I was at the front door using doggy sign language. I'm impressed because I can't train my dog to do anything. She opens the door and I introduce myself. While I'm speaking, she watches my lips and repeats everything I say in a low voice. I stutter and she gets hung up but keeps tracking. Her eyes move quickly from my lips to my eyes then back and her lips mimic mine when I stutter. I have experienced every imaginable reaction to a stutter, but this is a communication bridge I had yet to come across. I am rarely at a loss for words or a smartass comment, but in that moment I have no idea what to say, so I say, "I stutter."

Then her eyes open wide, worried she's offended me and she puts her hands in front of her mouth and wiggles her fingers like she's playing a flute. Suddenly I feel like Kevin Costner in *Dances with Wolves* trying to say "buffalo." I'm worried about insulting her, she's worried about insulting me and her dog is looking at us sideways like he wished he brought popcorn.

I shrug my shoulders, she says, "Stutter," making the gesture with her hand again and I nod, the universal sign for 'got it'. Turning my head to the street I point to my truck parked halfway between her and her neighbor's driveway and I ask if it's ok to park there. She says politely, "Please look at me when you speak." I feel like an idiot for my obvious blunder and repeat myself, now looking at her. The way she watches my lips triggers my stutter for some reason. I'm making *her* stutter and she's making *me* stutter. Jarred by that realization, I can't help but laugh at both of us and she joins me, laughing at our situation. She looks me in the eyes with a wide smile and says, "It's okay. No one lives next door."

From that point on, this deaf woman and I had an awesome conversation, laughing together over our shared challenges and enjoying a truly unique conversational experience.

It's okay to laugh at our differences. Coming from a place of good intentions or camaraderie, our differences can actually unite us.

I don't make fun of my stutter and am offended by jokes that do. *Spit it out!* or *C'mon, hurry up!* raises a fury in me that actually scares me. My emotional response to such taunts is something I need to work on, but I know I'll never be okay with it.

A stutter is not funny, but occasionally those situations a stutterer winds up in can be funny. Joking about something is not the same as joking about the person. Comedy is honesty in its purest form. If people are afraid to somehow offend you, can your relationship with them ever be honest?

Stutterers don't realize how self-conscious other people are about being polite to someone who is stuttering. The majority of people who are in a conversation with a stutterer are more worried about being rude or offensive than the stutterer is about giving them an inviting space to join in the conversation.

The fear of being mocked or insulted is an exaggerated fear with little chance of it becoming a reality. Being open, owning your stutter, and having a light-hearted attitude about it allows others to relax and get to know you.

Stutterers feel like they cannot express themselves. We know that the words we say are only 7% of what we communicate. We express 93% of our thoughts without words. So don't throw the baby out with the bath water. Open yourself up to *being* open. Typically, when people tell a stutter joke, they're trying to connect with you on a real and personal level. I love a good stutter joke, but it's actually hard to find one. A good joke captures the uncensored truth of a situation and not a preconception of the person. You can help our entire community overcome the common stereotype that we're all timid or nervous. Be ready to laugh at yourself, because you are no better or worse than the person who is trying so hard to connect with you that they feel compelled to tell you a stutter joke.

Bob and my boss are worried about offending me more than I'm concerned or sensitive to *being* offended. People are really cool, so I suggest that you let go of your self-involved narcissism, open up and get to know them.

I was terrified that I'd offended the deaf lady, and she was worried she offended me. What a waste of energy. People are not as easily offended as we think they are and I think it's time we let folks know that we're not as hyper-sensitive about our stutter as they may expect. Resiliency is the epitome of a stutterers journey.

22.
Blocking

Put all excuses aside and remember this:
You are capable.

~Zig Ziglar

It's no coincidence that "blocking" is a synonym for "frustration."
    Stuttering can be frustrating if you place more value on it than it actually holds. We are taught that stuttering is an involuntary disruption or blocking of speech. What we are not taught is that it's a disruption or blocking of speech, not the speech itself. We speak *with* a stutter; we do not speak *stutter*. It is separate from us, yet part of us, within us.

    Machines and computers stutter too, indicating a disruption in mechanical precision, electron flow, fine tuning, or timing. It's not a defect in the physical machine itself, merely an anomaly of consistent functioning. If you "stutter spoke" you would stutter inside your head, and you and I both know you don't stutter inside your mind as you formulate verbal expression.

Your brain formulates a fluent message, but what comes out of your mouth may belie that fluency with a stutter. Somewhere between the thought and muscle movements involved in producing speech there is an involuntary disruption.

This disruption causes blocking, and—trust me, I know from experience—blocking is frustrating. That's a given. But the obverse of that is that *frustrating is blocking*. I know; that sounds like razzle-dazzle logic. But which one is the cause and which one is the effect? That depends on which one can be manipulated by the other, doesn't it?

If you stutter, you become frustrated. If you're frustrated you stutter. Do they happen simultaneously? Is it a chicken before the egg kind of thing? Neither, it's a revolving door and you're stuck in it because you can't decide whether to stay in the building or go outside. Metaphorically, it's safe in the building. Climate controlled, security guards, and comfy couches. The weather is unpredictable outside, help is not readily available, and things can quickly become uncomfortable.

Any stutterer who has achieved any level of fluency through therapy or self-development will tell you that fluency does exist inside your comfort zone. Neither does success, love or happiness. Welcome to "Life," where progress only occurs by working through discomfort.

Your stutter frustrates you because you blame everything on it, and your frustration makes you stutter because you need something to blame.

You're spinning around in this revolving door, for years and years. If you go inside where it's comfortable, you feel safe but trapped. If you go outside where the wind blows unpredictably, you feel exposed to the elements.

Comfort and stuttering, or risk and improved fluency. This, my friends, is a choice only you can make. There is no amount of sympathy or safety inside to ease the feeling of being locked in a verbal prison, and there is no amount of ambition, invention, or achievement outside to buy a cure for stuttering.

Your level of fluency is in direct correlation to the confidence with which you stutter. The confidence with which you stutter is inverse to your fear of stuttering and your fear of stuttering is the direct product of the frustration that makes you stutter.

It's a classic "vicious circle": Stuttering causes frustration . . . which causes stuttering.

This is why fighting your stutter only makes it worse. If your stutter no longer frustrates you because you choose to own it, your body does not block it. It has no wall to hit and flows out of your mouth like water moving around rocks in a river. There will be ripples and bubbles in that water, but doesn't build up (become a block) anywhere. The water (your speech) may be bumped temporarily off course but it's not stopped. It becomes a variable, creates its own definition, becomes accented, not impeded.

At one time, when encountering certain verbal blocks, my entire body would lock up and my eyes would roll to the back of my head. I was fighting the tightening in my throat with my head and face muscles. It was an unconscious event, much like a seizure. I know stutterers who define the phenomenon of "blocking" as an involuntary phenomenon, reporting that it's not controllable, so they can't be "responsible" for the block.

That's not really a debate worth getting into, and if that's your take on blocking, you can own *that*. But I for one don't ask people who have not experienced something themselves for their opinions about how to do that thing. It's not too productive, in my opinion, to ask smokers for advice on how to quit smoking, ask obese people how to lose weight, or seek parenting advice from childless bachelors.

The first step toward fixing a problem is admitting you have a problem. If you cannot admit that you might not know the facts of lurking behind your problem, you can never learn how to fix it.

Tell the truth, be honest. Stop making excuses to feel sorry for yourself. Stop eating sympathy cookies and hoping everybody else will be there to support your physical and emotional needs.

Are you feeling uncomfortable? Good.

You need to step out of your comfort zone, because that's where fluency is. Fold up your blanky, give it back to your mom with a card that says thanks for everything, lace your combat boots up and let's go kick some ass.

Seriously, I've got your back. My name is on the cover of this book, so I'm am not some incognito troll telling you to think before you speak or admonishing you to "just stop stuttering." I am a father, son, brother, nephew, grandson, veteran, entrepreneur, lover, friend and human being who has lived and fought in the trenches of stuttering. I have been beaten, abused, attacked, loved, babied and sympathized for because I stutter. I speak with over 90% fluency and I haven't been to speech therapy since the sixth grade.

How did that happen?

Little by little. I learned the hard way because I'm a stubborn knucklehead who felt like his stutter was a special kind of stutter that no one understood.

You're probably wondering that if what I'm saying is true, why your parents or speech therapist don't tell you that. First of all, they probably don't stutter, so they don't know. If they don't stutter, they *can't* know. Secondly, they love you, so they're the last people who are going to tell you that you're acting like a victim. My mom thinks everything I write is the greatest thing she's ever read. My friends call me a great writer.

My editor says I'm prolific but I'm not great and probably has to take antacids by the third chapter because the entire second chapter was a four minute run-on sentence with no frickin' structure.

But guess what? It's not the responsibility of my mom or friends to do the uncomfortable job of calling me out, and it's not the responsibility of your parents or friends to tell you the painful truth. Putting that on them isn't fair. You're not in the third grade and your shitty finger painting is, truth be told, not good enough to be on the fridge.

Are you ready to roll, Soldier? Are you ready to stop being frustrated with your stutter and start being frustrated by the *reasons* you stutter? I don't know why you stutter, and until *you* know, discovering that "why" is your number one mission. I do know how to find out what fuels it, and once you find out the revolving door will stop and you'll have no choice but to go through it to the outside...or to step back from the reality it offers and stay cooped up, nice and safe and warm in your comfort zone.

The only way to find out what fuels your stutter is to figure out what you get from it. I don't mean the bad stuff, I mean what you gain from it. Attention, sympathy, a pass on altercation, financial support, a place to live, an excuse not to work hard or at all, an excuse to be a pothead, boozer or pill popper, hugs from Mommy, a car from Daddy, your place in the stuttering community, pity sex, a cover-up for co-dependency, nice guy/girl syndrome, insecurities, selfishness/narcissistic tendencies . . .

The list goes on forever, never ending (like some of my sentences, I know). I am not by any means accusing you of anything, and I know that you've never even considered this, so it's obviously not intentional on your part. I get that. All I want to do for you is to shed light on a dark little secret that has been kept from you by a part of you that operates with no distinction between right from wrong. If a machine stutters, it doesn't consciously do so to get attention from the technician. It runs off of a program, doing what it's told by algorithms and lines of code.

But now you're the genius hacker and this is your opportunity to rewrite the code. This may take some shadow work and you may have to go into the dark places of yourself that you don't feel particularly comfortable exploring. You may feel shame for never looking inside to find that grain of sand gumming up your machinery, but this isn't about guilt or shame or self-recrimination. This is about self-love and acceptance, not blame or punishment. You'll keep this private, and if you do it right, you'll confess it later because it feels good to be free from it but for now it's all about you. You're a hacker collecting private information which you will use to buy a brand new life.

It's very difficult to do this in the present tense, so think back in time. When you were a kid and would have given your right arm to not stutter what did you get from it? Did it feel good to be different, special, or unique? Could you blame bad grades or bad behavior on it? Did your parents spoil you or let you sleep in their bed because of it? There may be a multitude of "benefits" you got from stuttering, but they will all boil down to one.

You need to find that grain of sand, that one primary need in your life that was fulfilled by your stuttering. By identifying what need was met by stuttering, you can identify what it is you *still need today*. This isn't a bad thing, or a criticism of any kind. We all need stuff. Everybody grows up with needs that went unmet as children, and as adults we either overcome them unconsciously by trying achieve something else or we use manipulative tactics to somehow get what we need.

As a kid, I loved cuddling. I was a total cuddler, and as an adult I still wanted cuddles. I loved the feeling of physical affection and still do. In my relationships as a grown man I've unconsciously created strategies to receive physical affection. I'd display my "hurt" or appear "sad" so the caretaking nature of my partner would kick in and she'd be compelled to nurse me back to health. I was insecure and wanted to be held, so I would act like a four-year-old who'd had a bad dream.

When I finally realized this had been my self-soothing narcissistic tactic throughout my several personal relationships, I was embarrassed. Here I was, in my early thirties, and still needing cuddles. I had no reason to feel that way. Look, I still think cuddles are awesome. But manipulating people into giving cuddles is not. Just ask for the damned cuddles! Say it out loud: "Hey! I want some cuddles!"

No, this sort of honesty won't make you stop stuttering, but it *will* release your dependent attachment to the stutter. Once you're no longer attached to the stutter as a precursor to a reward, you can see it as an observer.

When I was younger, my mouth would get stuck open, my eyes would roll back and I'd momentarily lose physical control. I've meditated deeply on this and taken myself back to those disfluent episodes, recalling everything about that time in my life and what was going through my mind. Once I'd begun to speak, I'd lost all control over my body and couldn't stop the eye-rolling and twitching once it started. In recalling those episodes, I focused on what I'd done to overcome them. Over time, I learned to just . . . stop. Basic speech therapy, just stop. Breathe in, exhale slowly releasing the sound. I already knew I was supposed to do this, but I had to overcome the subconscious block before I could stop the physical one.

The first step is to stop.

Gain control by redirecting the block into the ground. Once momentum builds, inertia takes over and the energy goes up into your head and face. In other words, learn to stall the engine. Pushing the brakes and gas at the same time then releasing the brake to peel out a full sentence is how we learn to do it through desperation. Your throat is full throttle pushing out air but your vocal chords and jaw are locked, your eyes are just the tach gauge redlining.

I know you hate being told something so simple as stop and breathe, but *stop and breathe*. You may already do this out of habit, but you need to break the habit. Make it a conscious moment that *you control*. There will be withdrawal symptoms, but you have to *take control*. Taking control of your facial muscles is no different from learning to control any other muscle. Building your biceps or quads requires sets of repetitions performed with proper form. If you throw weights around using momentum to reduce the effort it takes to lift a weight without pain, there is simply no real muscle development at the end of the day. Tell your muscles that *you are in control* and slowly lift your words with proper form. It's the same as learning to ride a bike. You're going to fall and slip off the pedals, but once you experience the balance and the feel of coasting, you'll realize that the more relaxed you are and the more confidence you have, the easier it becomes to ride that bike.

I know that sounds corny, but it's the absolute truth. When you learn to stop a block, everything changes. It feels like the wind on your face when riding a bike. The basic fundamentals of speech therapy are effective, but they are only tools. They only work in the hands of a confident technician with the dexterity and fine motor skills needed to calibrate a machine by touch.

I know there are devices and therapies and drugs and surgeries that claim to help alleviate stuttering. I have not tried them, so I cannot comment on them. But from my experience, stuttering is a *fight for control*. I won the fight when I realized that my stutter was only a reaction to my own feelings and that the stutter itself had no desire or need to control. My stutter was not a living thing fighting me for control, and when I stopped fighting it, the blocks became less severe.

It happens in stages. You release any attachment that you might have towards the stutter and this separates it from your physical body and it becomes a thing, not a limb. You learn to stop. You understand that there is no need to continue and you realize that you can take your foot off the gas. Once you can effectively stop, you learn to feather the clutch. You become intimate with all the muscles in your throat and face. Touch them, massage them, practice moving every one of them. Teach yourself to relax through meditation and feel the energy in your body, learn how to move it to different body parts. Become familiar with yourself and love yourself. It's your body and it's depending on you to nurture it.

It is possible to become more fluent and even completely fluent. It is possible step outside, free yourself from frustration, and live a life overflowing with amazing, deep, and intimate conversations as a stutterer. Imagine sitting around a bonfire with a circle of friends and telling a funny story or approaching someone you're attracted to, and your stutter being an attractive feature. Imagine what it would feel like to be so free from the shame and frustration of stuttering that you intentionally hang onto a small part of it because it's a scar you're proud of, earned through your own badass courage and perseverance.

Take it from me: that's a great feeling.

23.
Fighting

Change does not roll in on the wheels of inevitability,
but comes through continuous struggle.
~Martin Luther King Jr.

People who stutter feel as if they are not taken seriously whenever they assert themselves verbally. When people argue, they're trying to make a point. When stutterers argue, they're trying to make a point without it becoming lost in blocks and repetitions. It becomes more about the fight to speak and to get past that damned block than about what they were trying to say in the first place. The stutterer finds himself arguing verbally with other people and internally with himself.

Imagine two people in a swimming pool having a conversation. One person is standing chest deep on the shallow end of the pool and one person is wading in the deep end. The person on the shallow end is grounded. The guy in the deep end is exerting energy simply staying afloat and keeping his head above water. The argument becomes heated, the grounded person speaks his mind standing straight, arms crossed. The guy in the deep end is trying to inhale enough air to keep treading water, gasping and spitting water out of his mouth while trying to make a point. The grounded person is solely focused on the argument and expressing an opinion. The guy in the deep end is struggling for air; lactic acid is saturating his muscles fibers, and he's swallowing water.

The guy in the deep end has two choices at this point: Swim to the shallow end or swim to the rim of the pool. Swimming to the shallow end will result in a physical confrontation with the other person. Swimming to the rim is essentially running away. This is the fight or flight mechanism we all have. A confrontation results in adrenaline coursing through our systems. Our minds assess the situation and we decide whether to fight, freeze, or run.

Stutterers tend to avoid confrontations for this very reason, but avoiding confrontation creates a sense of frustration and low self-worth. As a child I chose to run, as a young man I chose to fight. Both are ineffective, and here's why. Running can result in two outcomes. Either you escape the situation and create space between yourself and the confrontation, or you empower the aggressor and trigger their predatory instinct to give chase. If you are able to create space between you, you may be out of harm's way, but your self-esteem takes a hit. You're essentially reinforcing a belief that you're inferior. You've become prey. Your body language manifests this inner dialogue and you'll unconsciously appear week, never to be taken seriously. As a mature adult your persona and posture will be submissive. Success, love, and happiness are the products of a healthy sense of self-worth. None of these can coexist with an inferiority complex or a submissive mindset.

As a child, I ran from bullies. This empowered them to hurt me more seriously and more frequently. As a young man, I chose to fight, but this empowered them as well by giving them the ability to control my actions. I never left any confrontation feeling submissive, but I still felt inferior because I had been forced to react to the actions of someone else. In either scenario I was under the control of the aggressor. Whether I chose to run or fight, I was still forced to choose. My actions were reactions. I was a puppet and the bullies held the strings. Whether I won or lost a fight, I was still powerless to assert my own thoughts or choices.

Stuttering is simply an inability to voluntarily control your speech. Control is your superpower. You are a whole being with many parts. Learning to control one part affects all the others.

What did that person in the shallow end of the pool have that the guy treading water on did not? He had control. Why did he have control? Because he was grounded. He was standing on a solid surface with no need for an adrenaline rush, breathing freely with no need to flail around to merely maintain a presence.

My uncle was a martial arts instructor. I looked up to him, because he could handle himself in any situation with poise and presence. I joined his class and excelled. I learned to fight with precision and control. After a few years, I was able to strike an opponent when and where I chose to. I could control their body with my own by directing their attention to one hand and striking them with the other.

My class once made a trip to San Jose to train with an affiliated martial arts dojo. I was chosen to spar with a member of the host dojo who not only spoke fluently, but spoke too much. This kid hit at full speed during half-speed exercises and obviously enjoyed hurting people. His father was a high ranking instructor, which apparently gave him an unearned sense of superiority. My uncle was a high ranking instructor as well, and his students were equally skilled in striking as well as conducting themselves with restraint.

As we approached the center of the mat, we stood at attention and bowed, as dictated by martial arts tradition. I then stepped back with one foot, grounding myself with 80% of my weight on my back foot and 20% on my front foot. My hands were in front of me, stable but relaxed. I breathed in through my nose and out through mouth slowly.

The other kid jumped up and down, side to side and made funny faces. The referee said *go* and I stood still. The other kid moved around a lot but didn't strike as I crept forward maintaining my grounded posture. He began to strike without aiming and lost control of the situation by flailing a kick, striking nothing but air. I lifted my front leg, still grounded on my back leg, and he kicked my shin. He kicked it hard and it hurt. He was able to kick it hard because he directed all of his attention and body weight to the target. If it was to my core it would have been a devastating blow but it was only to my shin. He had put his full attention on one small part of me, leaving the rest of his body off balance, ungrounded and vulnerable.

My uncle always focused our lessons on balance and presence. I hadn't learned how to do cartwheel kicks in mid-air, but I knew how to stay within myself and defend against spinning cartwheel kicks like this kid was throwing at me with no power because he was thinking about his next move before completing the previous one. Halfway through his strikes his focus shifted to the next strike he had in mind, therefore taking power from his move of the moment. I took the hits to my arms and sides. He stepped back a few feet to catch his breath and stepped towards me again, now with his weight on his front foot. He had all his weight on the foot he should've left free to strike with, so knowing he could not move it, I retaliated. His arms dropped because he couldn't lift his leg without having to shift his full weight to his back leg. This was the second time he concentrated all of his focus on one part of me, and while his hands were lowered, I spun on my grounded foot, lifted my striking foot as I turned with a back kick and again he focused his effort on one small part of me. I never extended my leg, because I used the momentum of my spinning body to deliver a backhand that broke his nose. As he began to bleed, I stood there calmly balanced.

Remaining grounded is more effective in a confrontation than any fancy words, comebacks or making a point. If your stutter is severe, trying to talk your way out of anything is the equivalent of flailing your arms and legs or throwing a bunch of half powered karate strikes.

The fact is that half the time you're talking, you're concentrating on how to say the next word before finishing the previous one. Trying to make a point verbally while spitting out water and gasping for air or trying to find your best weight distribution is pointless. Being grounded mentally is a result of being mentally strong. In a job interview you don't talk straighter, you shoot straighter.

In a verbal altercation the same rules apply. Most arguments are two people talking over each other in a contest to see who can say the most words the fastest. It's a zero-sum game, and if you choose to play this game as a stutterer, you're putting all of your weight on your striking leg and leaving yourself completely exposed. If you remain grounded and stutter, your opponent will most likely concentrate all of their energy towards one small part of you, your stutter. If you have not owned your stutter this will be a devastating blow to your core. If you have come to terms with your stutter and accepted it as a part of you, it will be a kick to the shin. If they concentrate all of their focus and strength on your shin, they leave their face exposed.

It's practically one of nature's immutable laws: distract them and break their nose. It felt great watching that loud-mouth kid choke on his blood, until the big picture unfolded. I had the situation under my control. I could've struck him anywhere I wanted. I gave up my control and lost. This was not a bloodsport *kumite*, but a friendly points sparring match between neighboring karate clubs. My hit was illegal and he won by default. I had lost control, ignoring my mental balance, and instead of winning the match, I lost. I could have played with him all day, I could have just as easily hit his chest and won. I could have embarrassed him in front of everyone by maintaining my composure and sportsmanship. I could have given my mentor a victory and made him proud of me. Instead of maintaining my stature as an intelligent and disciplined fighter, I'd brought shame upon myself and my dojo.

You don't struggle in the deep end of the pool because you stutter. You're flailing and gasping because you're not grounded and have no self-control. A loss of self-control creates frustration. Frustration—as we now know—is a synonym for blocking.

The more accomplished I became at fighting, the less I fought. The more skills I learned, the less I needed them. People didn't harass me the way they once did and I was treated with more respect by strangers. I did not advertise my abilities and nobody knew I was a martial artist.

What changed? Why did people change? At our most primitive level, we are pack animals. Animals communicate very little by verbal sounds. The hierarchy of a pack is seen by an outside observer by body language and composure. The weaker members of the pack are often victims of the dominant members. The weaker members run from, physically submit, and cower before their dominant superiors. This behavior is how the dominant members recognize that they are superior. Humans have developed spoken language and generally choose to communicate verbally. But we still unconsciously communicate through body language. Your walk, posture and eyes can communicate whether you can hold your own in a physical or verbal confrontation before it happens. Being grounded is a choice and a skill that you develop by acquiring knowledge and discipline. An intelligent person does not play zero-sum games or argue pointlessly. He listens, observes and acknowledges. A skilled fighter does not brawl. He breathes, maintains his balance and holds back his punches

When you know that you can win a fight, you are less likely to fight because you have nothing to prove. This is communicated through your body language to others. Watch people make their way through a crowd. It is obvious who is scared of confrontation and who is not. If you fear confrontation, you're more likely to encounter it because your body language is inviting it. Your presentation to the external world is a reflection of your inner awareness. What you focus on is what you attract. If you focus on fear, you will attract things to fear. If you focus on stuttering, you will attract stuttering. If you focus on self-discipline and inner strength you will attract the skill to achieve it.

    This is one of those things that cannot be faked. Just like you can't fake confidence, you cannot fake being grounded. You have to do the work. To be a skilled fighter you have to practice each movement ten thousand times. Every muscle in your body must be able to transfer energy to the next without losing strength or accuracy. Your eyes must be trained to read the subtle "tells" and responses of another person, and you must learn to take a hit. A skilled debater must learn how to connect thoughts into words in such a way that an entire argument is made with as few words as possible.

    Asserting yourself as a stutterer is no different than other skills at use in a competitive environment. The more grounded person always has the upper hand. The person observing with cool detachment has a better understanding of the bigger picture than the person flailing. Stuttering can feel exactly like you're trying to speak while choking on water and flailing to keep your head above the surface gasping for air. You can swim to the shallow end, "shallow" being the operative concept, and still lose, regardless of the outcome.

Dog-paddle your way to the rim of the pool and sulk about how unfair life is or become a skilled swimmer. Remain calm and allow your body to be buoyant. Our bodies are programmed to fight, freeze, or run according to our psychological conditioning. If we always fight, the opponent will attack. If we always run, the opponent will pursue.

But what if we freeze? Of course, we can always play dead or just take the beating. But what if by "freezing" we simply embrace *stillness*? What if "freeze" is defined as *cool* and we learn to keep our cool? A skilled fighter doesn't attack or run. He bows, keeping his eye on his opponent while showing respect. He grounds himself, placing his weight on his back leg, maintaining poise and balance. He breathes slowly in through his nose and out through his mouth, supplying his mind and body with sufficient oxygen while remaining calm as adrenaline courses his body, readying muscles for action. He may take hits from an opponent but those will strike only non-vital targets like his stutter, and he does not waste excessive energy in a zero-sum effort, exchanging words for words.

Faking a strike is no different from asking a question. "Why are you angry?" You are in control of your leg and controlling their focus anywhere you want it.

Letting them hit a small part of you, your stutter, exposes their vulnerabilities. If they are willing to sacrifice their fighting stance, their point of view, to hit your shin then they have no argument and are fearful of your retort.

If their assault continues and you protect your core and remain composed, they will tire themselves out. They will back up to catch their breath and you can fake a strike again by asking a question.

Until this point, you have not thrown a single blow. You are in complete control of yourself and of your opponent. You have not expended any energy or taken a hit to any vital target. You can continue this for as long as it takes. You're conserving energy while they are wasting it. You're exposing them through their own actions and letting them show weaknesses. The more they talk, the less valuable their words become. Words are currency, egos are inflatable. Let them bankrupt themselves by verbal inflation.

Take the high road. Why lose the integrity you have built by diminishing your victory with immaturity. Don't let them win by default. When they are exposed and your hand is flying toward their face powered by centrifugal force, lower it and decrease speed. "I don't agree but I hear you."

Do not defend your stutter or acknowledge that they stoop so low as to address it. They already know they've lost once they've done that. The second they sacrifice their fighting stance to strike a shin, they and all who witness the action realize the transparency of their charade. They expose themselves as shallow and unskilled. A skilled fighter would never expose his face to attack a shin.

If you feel as if you are forced to tread water in the deep end of the pool because you stutter, who says you can't be there on a floaty casually sipping a pina colada?

24. Respect

When you start respecting yourself, what follows is control over your life.
~Suze Orman

I am at a level of fluency now that stuttering is no longer the issue. In my younger years, if I received bad service in a restaurant, someone was rude to me, or I felt mistreated in any way, I would just let it go, swallow my pride, pretend to ignore the hurt. But that pain would smolder inside of me and eventually reveal itself as what can only be described as "a bad attitude." I knew that if I reacted to the hurt at the moment—like asking a waiter to check the inaccurate addition on a dinner tab—I would only bring attention to myself. Even when a fluent person takes a questioning or challenging tone in public, people react and take notice. When a stuttering, sputtering, blocking speaker asks the same question or offers even a remotely confrontational or contradictory comment, it has the potential to become a true social spectacle.

Just imagine it. What if . . .

You're at a hotel check-in desk and they've lost your reservation. The lobby is crowded and there are people impatiently in line behind you and checking in beside you. You've made the online reservation, they already have your credit card information, and you have your confirmation printed out and in your hand. You're in the right, but the officiously-snotty desk clerk is blowing you off and looking to the next person in line. It's one of those situations where the squeaking wheel gets the grease.

The fact is, the hotel overbooked for the night, and whoever fights for a room the loudest and most assertively gets one. What do you do?

All your life, everything you've gotten in such circumstances has been limited by your ability to speak up for it and you've rarely been given exactly what you wanted or needed. You've always slouched, your chest tightened, and you've sucked it up. Then you've logged onto a social media stutterers group and bitched about how you never get dinner orders the way you really want them. You've always wanted cinnamon sprinkles on that latté, but you can't have cinnamon sprinkles because you can't say "cinnamon."

So now, standing in that hotel check-in line, you're throwing a tantrum internally ready to go online and complain loudly about this lousy hotel service. But to complain online, you need a wi-fi connection, and you can only have one if you get a room...which this silly desk clerk is telling you is "unfortunately unavailable.

So here you stand at the counter, the clerk calling "next," and you have no hotel room with diminishing prospects of getting one. Take a breath and think back to the Sixth Grade when your turn was coming up to read in front of the class. What did you do then? Ask to go to the lavatory to avoid the entire ordeal? Didn't the teacher deny you a hall pass until you stood up and read from the textbook. Didn't those kids laugh at you as you squeaked through a paragraph, your eyes rolling, your tongue curling into a ball?

So what do you do now? Do you firmly place your palms on the counter, maintain your balance and composure, stand up straight and look this minimum-wage desk clerk flunky squarely in the eye as you take a deep breath and then calmly intone "I-I-I reserved this room a month ago. I-I-I need to speak with your manager"?

That's exactly what you do. Yes, you're going to feel everyone look at you, you might even turn red and you sure as hell will piss off the desk clerk (who—if you hold your ground—will begin to tremble). This may seem trivial or hypothetical, but it's not. It's purely existential. It's about *who you are as a* person.

You want fluency? Then stand up straight with your hands spread on the counter, look them in the eyes and say what you have to say, however you say it. Don't back down no matter what they say or who's watching. You can bitch about being laughed at in middle school, or while hating your cinnamon-less lattés for the rest of your life . . . or you can stand up for yourself physically and verbally.

Moments such as these are your opportunities to grow and to succeed, and you have a responsibility to yourself, to fellow stutterers—to me for writing this book—to seize upon these opportunities to *suck it* up and spit out exactly what you mean, no matter how long it takes to say it, no matter how many syllables you have to repeat, no matter how many eyeballs stare at you, no matter how many impatient sighs you hear.

I know that what I'm saying here may be sacrilege to the traditional "community" of stutterers who practice the fine art of word selection, avoidance of confrontation, and always nodding in silent agreement when we don't agree at all. But where does that get any of us stutterers?

The back of the room, that's where. Afraid to speak our minds, too timid to raise our hands, afraid to sit in the front row for fear of being "called on."

Screw that. You didn't get your eggs the way you like them or your six-dollar coffee the way you want it? Well, what do you expect? If you can't muster the fortitude to stutter in front of a cashier, you will never achieve any level of fluency or personal happiness. What are we doing as a "community" when our predominant complaint is about how the 17-year-old kid behind a counter might react when we have difficulty responding to her asking *How can I help you?*

As a child my stutter exiled me from the tribe. As an adult only I can exile myself. I am not a timid, weak or submissive stutterer. I am a professional, confident and secure stutterer.

Don't get me wrong: I have nothing but respect for the organizations devoted to stuttering. They are doing their part and doing it well. I'm speaking to you, the individual. The way you carry yourself and conduct business on a day-to-day basis is paramount not only for yourself, but for the kid on the playground who got socked in the jaw today because our culture sees stuttering as a sign of weakness.

What you have to say is not worth repeating. You said it fine the first time. If someone is impatient because you need more time to speak, how is that your problem?

Oh...wait. It's *not your problem*.

Take your time, say what you need to say in a civilized tone and move on. Every time you run to the bathroom when it's your turn to read in class, you are reinforcing in your subconscious that you *want to stutter*. All you're doing is reinforcing a self-fulfilling prophesy and you *will* stutter more. Every time you stand your ground you are you are telling your subconscious that the stutter is not necessary.

Take it from me. Standing your ground is worth it.

Tough Love

25.
The Bottom Line

What you get by achieving your goals is not as important as what you become by achieving your goals.
~Thoreau

I will fight on any platform for any stutterer, be it a debate or bare knuckles. I will not, however, defend a stutterer who dishonors those who have fought for our equality by portraying us as disadvantaged. We are not subjugated, submissive, or subpar on any level of the economic or social sphere. We are CEO's, politicians, lawyers, scientist, artist and history makers. We will not be defined by Hollywood or confined to the substratum of society. We are parents, caretakers and lovers. We are creators of great works, leaders of industries and a force of unfathomable resiliency.

Yes, I'm a stutterer. And I'm so much more.

I know you are, too.

Through the centuries, stutterers have faced discrimination and brutality. Tongues have been cut from peoples' mouths, brains have been sliced open and exorcisms performed. Over the course of a thousand years, stutterers have fought tooth-and-nail for the right to merely exist without the fear of mutilation or exile. Hollywood has made millions stigmatizing our speech disorder by portraying characters who are either intellectually challenged or cowardly. Stutterers are accused with false charges of intoxication, falsifying statements because they seem nervous or suspected of having a mental disorder.

I am in no way denying that discrimination does not or has not occurred. My intent is not to belittle the victims of these atrocities or those fighting for my right to compete on a level playing today.

In our online age where information is at our fingertips, we have an unlimited supply of resources. Speech therapy is free, support is readily available and associations, foundations, and organizations lead the charge in our battle to coexist as equals. Anti-discrimination laws protect us from flagrant violations of our rights. Society's dismay for bullies favors the underdog and we benefit from that.

To use our stutter as an excuse to fail is to say that stutterers *are* failures. To blame any addiction, abuse, or narcissistic behavior on our stutter is to say that stutterers are addicts, abusers and narcissists. To not reach your highest potential is a personal choice. To blame your stutter for your lack of ambition is to say that stutterers are inadequate. Society is shifting into a model of tolerance and acceptance. Our success as stutterers and perseverance in the face of adversity reinforces this shift. One day, the 3rd Grader who stutters will be seen as gifted instead of disadvantaged because those who blazed the trail before him as a collective became leaders of industries.

We get anxious and concerned when we take too long to make our conversational points or when we have difficulty ordering at a drive through. Our feelings get hurt if someone blinks upon introduction. These are petty complaints and fundamentally disrespectful to our community. Our inability to fully express ourselves verbally is not a restraint but a catalyst for creativity. In truth, spoken words are the cheapest of currencies. Our capacity to impact business, art, government, and the world at large is defined not by our utterances, but by our actions.

What we do in life is really all that matters.

Tough Love

Work hard.

Love harder,

Tough Love

About the Author

A native Californian, Shane Chapa served with the U.S. Army in the Middle East. He later worked as a licensed contractor and now calls Phoenix, Arizona home.

With a love of words and story-telling skills inspired by a 1st place prize in his 6th-grade statewide writing contest, Shane believes in connecting with his readers on the most vulnerable and sometimes painfully candid levels.

When he's not on job sites, sharing his thoughts via his online blog, or working on his next book, this proud father of two hikes the rugged mountains surrounding Phoenix, gathering the inspiration and strength to take his writing to "the next level."

Shane is available for private consultations and for compelling speaking engagements where he shares the tactics, methods, and mindset behind his personal fulfillment and success while living with a lifelong speech impediment.

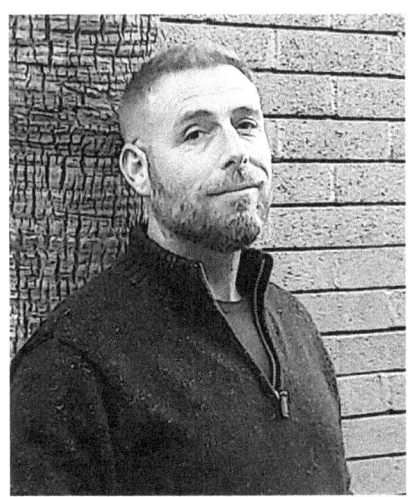

toughlovestutter@gmail.com

Chapa Communications
24 W. Camelback Rd., ste. A-218
Phoenix, AZ 85013

www.ingramcontent.com/pod-product-compliance
Lightning Source LLC
Chambersburg PA
CBHW071401210526
45465CB00001B/194